MOLOY'S

Evaluation of the Pelvis in Obstetrics

Third Edition

MOLOY'S

Evaluation of the Pelvis in Obstetrics

Charles M. Steer

M.D., Med.Sc.D., F.A.C.S., F.A.C.O.G.

Professor of Clinical Obstetrics and Gynecology
College of Physicians and Surgeons
Columbia University
and
Attending Obstetrician and Gynecologist
Presbyterian Hospital

Third Edition

PLENUM MEDICAL BOOK COMPANY
NEW YORK AND LONDON

Library of Congress Cataloging in Publication Data

Moloy, Howard Carman, 1903-
    Moloy's Evaluation of the pelvis in obstetrics.

    First ed. published in 1951 under title: Clinical and roentgenologic evaluation
of the pelvis in obstetrics.
    Includes bibliographical references and index.
    1. Pelvis—Radiography. 2. Obstetrics. I. Steer, Charles M. II. Title. III Title:
Evaluation of the pelvis in obstetrics. [DNLM: 1. Labor complications. 2. Pelvi-
metry. WQ310 M728c]
RC527.M64 1975   618.2   75-2208
ISBN 978-1-4757-0270-5   ISBN 978-1-4757-0268-2 (eBook)
DOI 10.1007/978-1-4757-0268-2

Foreword

THE prediction of the probability of the safe passage of the fetus through the birth canal is the primary function of the attendant at the start of labor. The means of determining the relative size of the fetal head and the internal diameters of the pelvis have therefore been the objects of deep concern down through the centuries.

Manual techniques of clinical evaluation of cephalo-pelvic relations reached their peak a generation or two ago. A massive nomenclature existed with respect to pelvic planes and diameters. To these were related various positions, attitudes, stations, and synclitisms of the fetal head. Measurements depended on digital efforts to explore the interior and on dubious implications drawn from external pelvimetry. The mechanisms of labor, as it might occur under the innumerable possible pelvic measurements and fetal orientations, were the subject of hours of student drilling and remained a lifelong preoccupation of the most seasoned specialist.

The increasing safety of cesarean section somewhat mitigated the consequences of error. When a borderline internal conjugate was digitally determined, a trial labor might be permitted with the assurance that an ultimate solution was in reserve. Mistakes of two kinds persisted, however. On the one hand, trial labor might be permitted to continue too long and, with penicillin not yet discovered, a delayed cesarean section

could be perilous. Alternately, to be on the safe side, many un-
necessary elective sections might be carried out.

The development of an accurate method for determining
pelvic measurements became possible with the elaboration of
roentgenographic techniques. The work of Howard Moloy and
William Caldwell, begun in 1929, was based on the use of the
x-ray stereoscope. It set in motion a whole series of studies which
led to a revolution in the evaluation of the pelvis and in the pre-
dictability of the course of labor.

Caldwell and Moloy began with the devising of precise
methods for the measurement of critical—but digitally inacces-
sible—diameters of the pelvis. With the figures so obtained in
hand, there became possible a synthesis in the form of the recognition of four basic types of pelves, the normal, "gynecoid," as
well as the somewhat atypical "android," "anthropoid," and
"platypelloid" forms. The immediate result of the new classification was the abandonment of a pathologic etiology, as implied
in such terms as "rachitic pelvis," and the acceptance of the idea
that the variations were in general congenital or environmental.

All of this was, however, only a beginning. The new techniques, and the accurate information on size and shape of the
pelvis they provided, made necessary a complete review of the
mechanism of labor. The position of the fetal head and a fair
estimation of its essential dimensions were soon added to the
available data. There then followed years of study during which
statistics were collected from actual observations to assist the
obstetrician in his prognoses and in his decisions on how to con-
duct the course of labor under a wide variety of circumstances.

Much of the knowledge derived from these earlier clinical
studies was utilized in the preparation of the first and second
editions of this work. In the present volume there has been
added important new material on the management of breech
delivery. Here certain special technical difficulties in measurement exist, since the fetal head cannot be visualized in immediate relation to the pelvic diameters, and the continued higher

perinatal mortality in cases with breech presentation renders this a problem of the greatest importance.

In obstetrics, as in all clinical medicine and indeed in all science, the area of the greatest concentration of research interest changes from year to year. Particular attention is now directed to the fetus, with various monitoring systems, and to the newborn, with intensive care units for the jeopardized. Although not all the handicaps borne by the fetus and the newborn are due to prolonged labor or traumatic delivery, a substantial portion certainly are. For the prevention of these, the early recognition of cephalo-pelvic disproportion is essential. The x-ray evaluation of the obstetrical pelvis may now be regarded as a mature science and the proper use of these techniques remains one of the essentials of the competent practitioner.

HOWARD C. TAYLOR, M.D.
Professor Emeritus of
Obstetrics and Gynecology
College of Physicians and Surgeons
Columbia University

Preface to the Third Edition

In the years between the publication of the first and second editions of this work devoted to evaluation of the pelvis in obstetrics, further studies devoted to the recognition of disproportion were carried out. This later work was begun by Dr. Moloy and the present author, and was completed by the present author after Dr. Moloy's untimely death. These new studies allowed a complete presentation of up-to-date knowledge of the pelvis in obstetrics, which was first detailed in the second edition and appears unchanged in the present volume.

The various types of pelves are described; methods of recognizing them are presented; and the effect of pelvic shape upon the mechanism of labor is discussed. Measurement of the space available in the pelvis is described, and the outcome of labor in varying degrees of disproportion is detailed. With this information, it then becomes possible to estimate the probable course of labor from the mechanical point of view, and also to determine the best and safest way of managing those cases in which progress is arrested. In order to present the management of pelvic arrest, the very short section on forceps in the first edition was replaced in the second edition by a section on the influence of pelvic shape in the management of obstructed labor, and breech presentation is considered in a section new to this third edition.

This book is not designed to replace standard textbooks on obstetrics. The obstetric forceps and their use, breech delivery, and other features of obstetrics are best studied in a comprehensive text. This very specialized volume is designed to prepare the operator so that the proper method of delivery may be chosen in each individual case.

The classification of pelves is given in some detail. This is necessary because such variations do exist, and some method of naming them is required. The *really important* feature, however, lies in the influence of these variations upon the mechanism of labor. Whether the forepelvis is "android" or "anthropoid" in type is not nearly so important as recognition of the fact that the forepelvis is *narrow*, that the space available is less because of this, and that management of labor will consequently be different.

CHARLES M. STEER, M.D.

Contents

Section I

Section II

Section III

Section IV

Section V

Section I

General Morphology of the Pelvis

In this monograph an attempt is made to describe the variations in the female pelvis which are of obstetrical significance, to correlate these with their effect upon labor, and to indicate how, by clinical and roentgenological methods of examination, the various abnormalities may be recognized.

In the ideal obstetrical department there should be a room set aside for the routine study of the pelvic architecture. It should contain mounted pelves or pelvic models on which can be demonstrated the pelvic planes and diameters and which can be used to illustrate labor mechanisms. It should also be equipped with adequate viewing cabinets for the study of the roentgenological films. With such facilities it becomes at once a study center and the place where clinical and roentgenological data can be correlated in each individual case under review. It is here that obstetrical prognoses are made and lines of treatment discussed.

ANALYSIS OF PELVIC SHAPE

The first essential in studying anatomic variations in the pelvis is to have a clear appreciation of the shape and size of the normal pelvic cavity and of the criteria used to define normality and departures therefrom. A scheme for such study

1

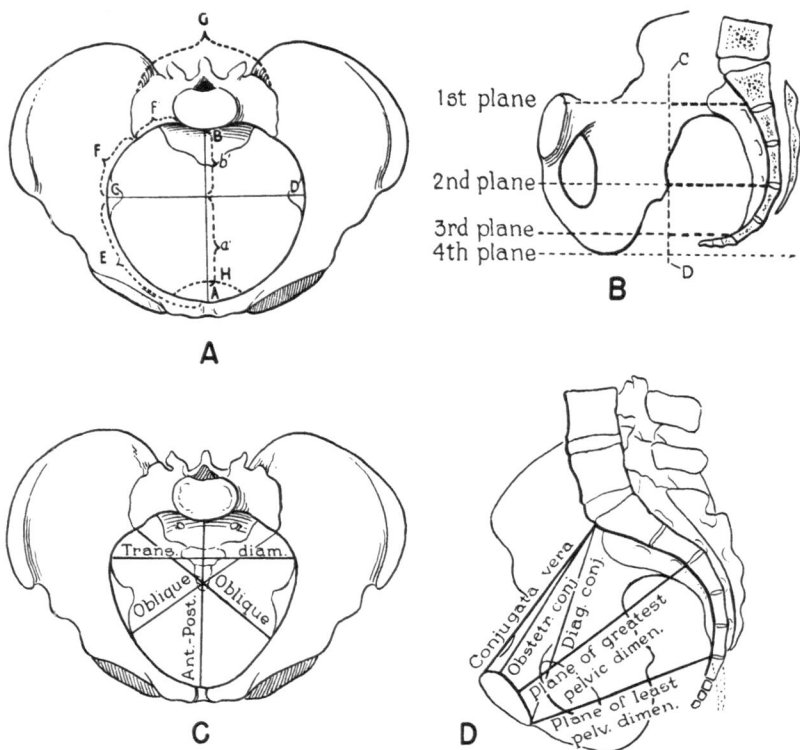

Figure 1. Scheme of analysis of pelvic morphology: A, inlet view; B, lateral view. Conventional pelvic planes and diameters: C, inlet view; D, lateral view.

is illustrated in Fig. 1, A,B. This scheme is a departure from the conventional division of the pelvic cavity, illustrated for comparison in Fig. 1, C,D. In the latter the pelvis is divided by imaginary planes which diverge from the short symphysis to the long sacrum. This concept assumes that the true pelvic cavity is shorter in front than behind. The study of roentgenograms from patients in labor has shown, however, that this concept is not true. The true pelvic cavity is comparable to a cylinder with straight side walls or to a parallelogram as deep in front as behind. The head descends much like a piston, until it reaches a level at which it can move forward under the subpubic arch. A study of the conventional diameters illustrated in Fig. 1, D, indicates why oblique sagittal diameters are not significant. The head may descend below one origin of an oblique diameter before it is confronted with the other situated at a lower level. The conventional oblique inlet diameters illustrated in Fig. 1, C, are not used in roentgenologic diagnosis.

There exist 4 planes parallel to each other, all of which are perpendicular to the coronal plane CD. The first plane to be located is the coronal plane CD (Fig. 1, A,B) which passes through two fixed and easily identified diameters:

1. The widest transverse diameter of the inlet.

2. The interspinous diameter (the line joining the posterior aspects of the ischial spines).

To locate this plane in skeletal pelves place the thumb tips at the origin of the widest transverse diameter. Look through the inlet from above and rotate the pelvis until these two diameters are situated one above the other in the same coronal plane as illustrated in Figs. 2 and 3. The posterior aspect of each ischial spine is easily identified, but the precise points of origin of the widest transverse diameter are sometimes more difficult to locate. By trial and error, it is possible to identify the origin of this diameter, selecting arbitrary points at the inlet, where the iliopectineal lines begin to converge posteriorly toward the sacroiliac synchondrosis and anteriorly toward the

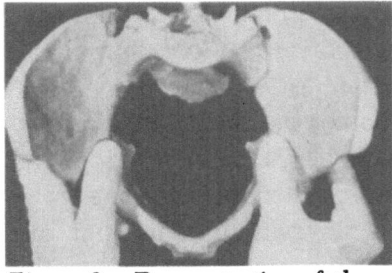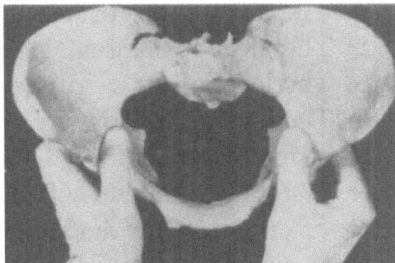

Figure 2. Demonstration of the coronal plane through the inlet in two different pelvic types.

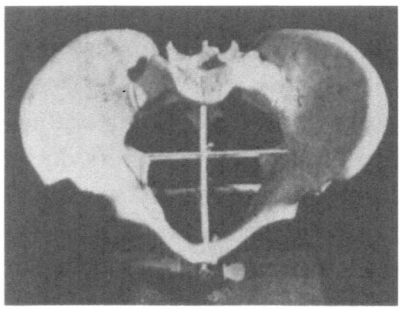 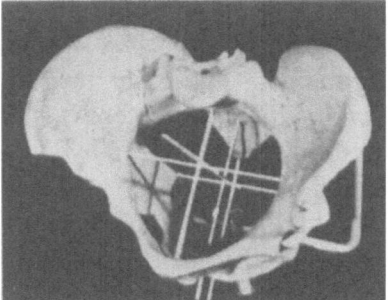

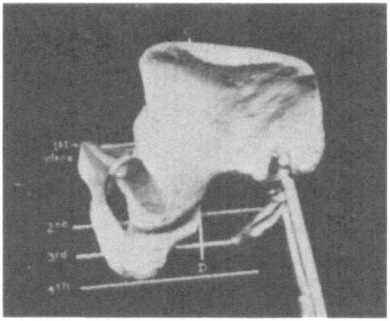

Figure 3.   Inlet, oblique, and lateral views of a pelvic model, to show
the pelvic planes and diameters.

forepelvis. This coronal plane divides the true pelvic cavity
into an anterior and posterior segment.

The description of variations at lower levels in the true
pelvis is aided by the use of horizontal planes. These planes
are drawn at right angles to the coronal plane CD (Fig. 1, B)
and are situated at the following levels:

1. The level of the widest transverse diameter at the inlet
2. The level of the ischial spines
3. The level of the sacral tip
4. The level of the lowest portion of the ischial tuberosities

The significant sagittal diameter at the inlet refers to the
anteroposterior diameter of the first horizontal plane. The
points of origin of this diameter, at the symphysis in front and
the sacrum behind, are selected entirely upon the basis of the
right angle relationship of the diameter to the coronal plane

and vary in position slightly with each pelvis (Fig. 3). The conjugata vera or true conjugate diameter is usually defined as a line extending from the promontory of the sacrum to the upper posterior aspect of the symphysis. In most instances this diameter corresponds in length with the anteroposterior diameter of the first horizontal plane as above defined.

There are exceptions to this rule, however, and two extreme examples are illustrated in Fig. 4. In one (Fig. 4, A), the promontory, situated above the level of the first plane, overhangs the posterior pelvis and causes a reduction in the length of the true conjugate diameter. The sacrum has a marked concavity with a backward inclination. For this reason, the anteroposterior diameter of the first horizontal plane is longer than the true conjugate diameter. This situation may occur in flat pelves. The head may negotiate the short true conjugate diameter by asynclitism, provided the promontory is high with respect to the level of the top of the symphysis pubis. The other extreme example illustrated in Fig. 4, B, reveals a true conjugate diameter which is longer than the anteroposterior

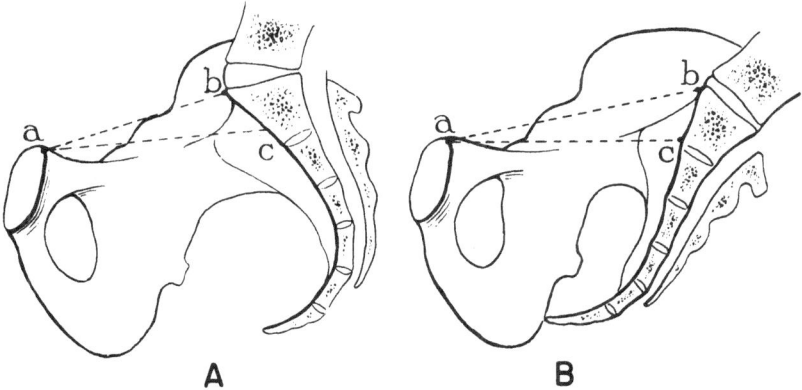

A   B

Figure 4. Relationship of true conjugate diameter to the anteroposterior diameter of the first horizontal plane. Exaggerated examples are illustrated. A, A short, true conjugate diameter (a–b) associated with a longer anteroposterior diameter of the first horizontal plane (a–c). B, A long, true conjugate diameter (a–b) associated with a shorter anteroposterior diameter of the first horizontal plane (a–c).

diameter of the first plane because the promontory is high and is displaced backward due to the presence of a forward sacral inclination. A study of these two diagrams will show that a short true conjugate diameter may not be as significant as a short anteroposterior diameter of the first horizontal plane because the latter diameter originates from bony points situated at the same level.

The so-called fixed relationship of the coronal plane is demonstrated only under the conditions illustrated in Figs. 2 and 3. It cannot be demonstrated in roentgen films by roentgen technics which utilize oblique inlet views. In the Thoms semisitting position with the inlet plane parallel to the film, by chance, the target may be centered over the midpoints of the widest transverse and interspinous diameters and so demonstrate the coronal plane as illustrated in Figs. 2 and 3.

Variations in the point of intersection of the widest transverse diameter and the anteroposterior diameter of the inlet modify the lengths of the anterior and posterior sagittal diameters. This variation is reflected in the length of the ilium over the sacrosciatic notch between the origins of the widest transverse diameter and the sacroiliac synchondrosis. Extremes in variations in two human pelves are illustrated in Fig. 2.

A study of the pelvis through the inlet locates the position of the widest transverse diameter and shows the shape of the anterior and posterior pelvic segments. Directly below the widest transverse diameter of the inlet, the interspinous diameter is observed at the level of the second parallel plane. At lower levels, the encroachment of the lower sacrum behind and below the ischial spines at the third plane may be noticed. At the lowest level of the pelvis, or fourth plane, the "widest transverse diameter of the outlet" may be readily identified. This diameter gives the width of the outlet and is a better obstetric term than the usual "intertuberous diameter."

In the lateral view of the pelvis the length of the true conjugate diameter, the shape of the sacrosciatic notch, and the curvature and inclination of the sacrum may be appreciated.

The lateral view reveals to advantage the region behind and below the ischial spines.

The side walls and the subpubic arch determine the available transverse space at lower levels. The subpubic arch varies in size and shape and these variants in turn must be associated with the widest transverse diameter of the outlet and the degree of convergence or divergence of the pelvic side walls.

SEXUAL DIFFERENCES IN PELVES

Photographs of inlet, lateral and subpubic arch views of the typical male and female pelvis are shown in Fig. 5.

In the male, when the inlet is studied with the widest transverse diameter and the interspinous diameter visually superimposed from above, the posterior segment appears flat in shape. The sagittal diameter of the posterior segment is short. The origin of the widest transverse diameter is separated from the sacroiliac synchondrosis by a short section of the ilium. The sacrosciatic notch, at a lower level, is narrow, and the anterior edge of the first sacral vertebra is usually flat. The anterior segment reveals a narrow retropubic angle. The iliopectineal lines passing backward from the symphysis are straight as compared to the female pelvis and give a wedge-shaped appearance to the inlet.

The posterior segment of the female pelvis shows greater length between the origin of the widest transverse diameter and the sacroiliac synchondrosis. The sacrosciatic notch, at a lower level, shows greater width. The anterior edge of the first sacral vertebra shows a definite transverse curvature, which increases the length of the posterior sagittal diameter at the inlet. The anterior segment is well rounded with a wide retropubic angle. The iliopectineal lines passing backward from the symphysis to the widest transverse diameter are curved to correspond to the wide retropubic angle. The shape of the two segments of the inlet combines to give a slightly ovoid to round appearance.

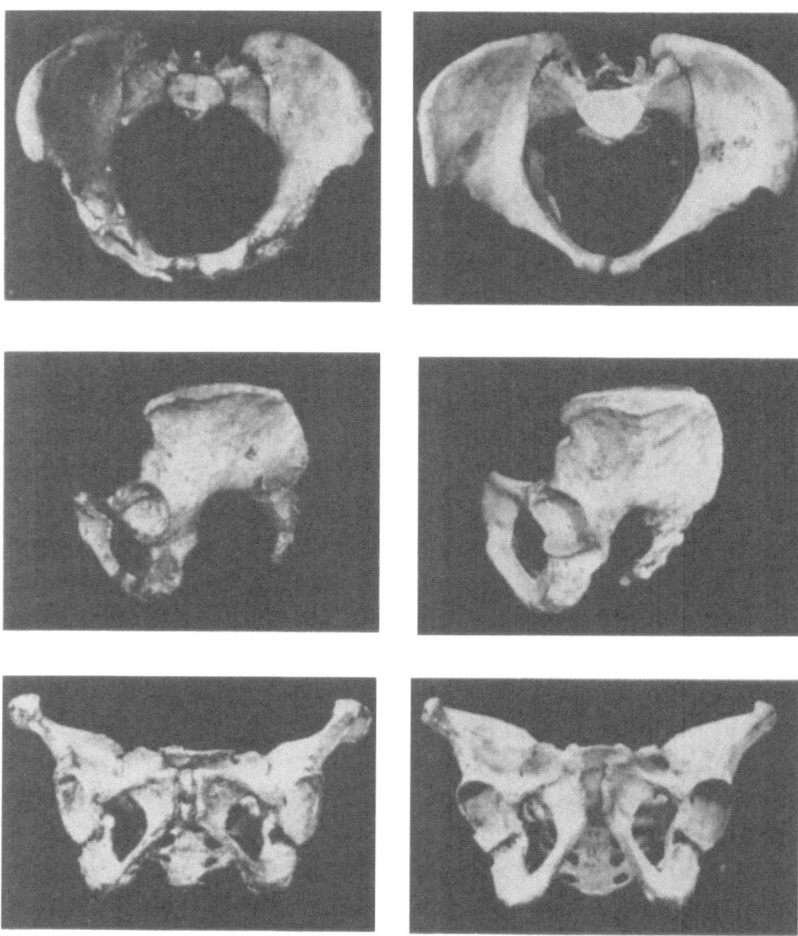

Figure 5.   Inlet, lateral, and subpubic arch views of typical male (right) and female pelves.

The lateral view of the male pelvis shows the character-istic long, narrow sacrosciatic notch. Also, the ilium extends downward to form at least one-third of the posterior boundary of the notch, before curving posteriorly to the posterior inferior iliac spine. In the female, the apex of the notch is wide and the ilium passes directly backward to the posterior iliac spine without contributing noticeably to the posterior boundary of the notch. These important sex characteristics in and above the sacrosciatic notch are illustrated in Derry's[1] diagram (Fig. 6). The lateral view of the male and female pelvis and Derry's diagram bring out another minor sex difference: the crest of the ilium is rectangular in the male and circular in the female.

The sacrum in the male usually shows a forward inclina-tion, causing a shortening of the posterior sagittal diameters at the level of the second and third horizontal planes. In the female, the sacrum is distinctly backward, causing a lengthen-ing of the lower posterior sagittal diameters. The subpubic arch and pubes reveal marked sex differences. In the male, the symphysis is long and narrow. The subpubic arch is narrow

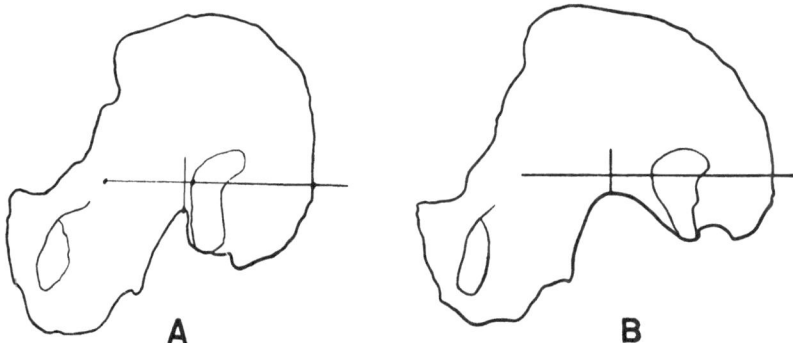

A   B

Figure 6. The distance from the apex of the notch on the iliopec-tineal line to the sacroiliac synchondrosis is shorter in the male than in the female. For this reason the posterior sagittal diameter at the inlet be-hind the widest transverse diameter is shorter in the male and in android types than in gynecoid and anthropoid forms. A, Male. Compare the area of sacroiliac contact. In the male this is perpendicular, giving a forward inclination to the sacrum. B, Female. In the female the articular surface slopes backward because the sacrum has a backward inclination. (From Derry, D. E.: J. Anat. & Physiol., Vol. 46, 1923.)

and the free edges of the pubic rami are straight or wedge-shaped, giving a "Gothic" arch effect. The pubic rami appear to originate from the lower medial aspect of each pubic bone. The side walls of the anterior segment converge to cause marked reduction in the length of the interspinous and intertuberous diameters. This gives a funnel-shaped appearance to the lower forepelvis.

In the female, the pubes are short and broad. The pubic rami are well curved, giving a "Norman" arch effect. The angle of the arch is wide or average in size. The pubic rami in the female appear to originate from the lower lateral aspect of the symphysis. The pelvic side walls are straight and the interspinous and intertuberous diameters are wide.

Male and female pelves also differ in pelvic depth. The depth is measured on a line joining the brim and the ischial tuberosities. There is an average difference of approximately 1 cm., as determined from Todd's skeletal material of known sex. The male pelvis also shows heavier bones than the female pelvis. However, a study of the roentgenograms of male pelves will occasionally reveal examples of delicate bones and other gynecoid characteristics, as for instance a wide retropubic angle and straight pelvic side walls.

CLASSIFICATION OF PELVES

Anatomic and roentgenologic studies have shown that variations in the size and shape of the pelvis occur more frequently than was hitherto suspected. More recent studies have gone far in appraising the significance of these variations upon the mechanism of labor. The chief differences in opinion now concern the correct classification of these variations.

In the classification proposed by such authorities as Michaëlis, Litzmann, Tarnier, Budin, Schauta, Breus and Kolisko, and others, some wholeheartedly accepted the principle that an obstetric classification should be arranged according to the etiology of the factors which caused the distortion. They attempted to fit abnormalities of doubtful origin into appropriate subgroups. Others, recognizing the prevalence of pelvic abnormalities for which no known explanation existed, introduced such morphologic terms as "flat-nonrachitic pelvis," "funnel pelvis," or "generally contracted type." Although Michaëlis and Litzmann favored the morphologic school of thought, the preconceived methods and lack of knowledge prevented the general acceptance of their views. Anatomists and anthropologists have always considered form in the study of unknown skeletal material. Stein (1825) distinguished four groups:

1. Elliptic, with the greatest diameter anteroposterior
2. Round
3. Elliptic, with the greatest diameter transverse
4. Blunt heart-shaped

Turner,[2] in 1885, proposed a morphologic classification based upon the relationship of the transverse and anteroposterior diameters of the inlet. He divided pelves into three groups:

1. Dolichopellic, in which the conjugata vera is greater than the transverse diameter.

2. Mesatipellic, in which the conjugata vera and transverse diameter are of equal length.

3. Platypellic, in which the conjugata vera is shorter than the transverse diameter.

Thoms[3] has recently revised Turner's classification and has added a fourth group—the brachypellic form. Thoms classifies the pelvis according to these four types (dolichopellic, mesatipellic, brachypellic and platypelloid) by the use of the pelvic index aided by visual inspection of the inlet view.

The limitation of the pelvic index as an indicator of shape is shown by the fact that the variations in the index for android and gynecoid types are similar. This point is illustrated in Fig. 7, which shows that the pelvic index does not reveal the presence of such android features as, for instance, a narrow

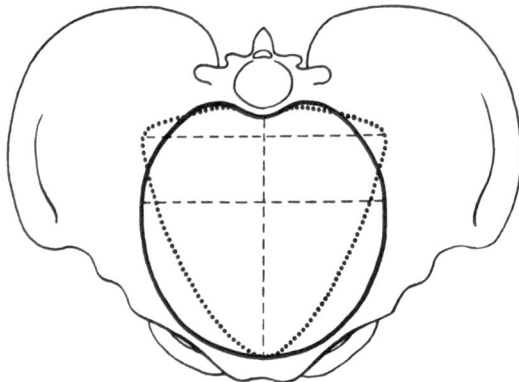

Figure 7. A diagram to show that android and gynecoid types may
have a similar pelvic index.

forepelvis, nor does it indicate the variable point of intersection
of the widest transverse diameter and the anteroposterior diameters at the level of the first plane of the inlet.

The pelvic index, however, is useful to indicate trends in
the extremes in shape either for the longish oval or anthropoid
component, or for a transverse oval or flat component. This
fact has practical value in placing a pelvis in the anthropoid
and intermediate anthropoid groups, or in the flat and intermediate flat forms, using inlet measurements as obtained by
roentgen pelvimetry.

Type	Range of Variation for AP Diameter	Range of Variation for Widest Transverse Diameter
Anthropoid and Intermediate Anthropoid Types	11.5 — 12.5 cm	11.5 — 13.5 cm
Gynecoid and Android	10.5 — 11 cm	12.5 — 13.5 cm
Flat and Intermediate Flat	9 — 10.5 cm	12 — 14 cm

The classifications of Weber, von Stein, and Turner made
no provisions for the intermediate forms.

During the early part of this century, anthropologists made
a number of observations not fully appreciated by obstetricians.
Wood Jones and Elliot Smith,[4] during excavations in Nubia in

1906, found many extreme masculine types of female pelves. Derry, Straus, and others have described masculine characteristics helpful in determining the sex of unknown skeletal material. Recent anthropologists—Hrdlicka, Todd, Hooton, Schultz, Shapiro, and others—are convinced that the variations in pelves are too complex to be grouped in the simplified classifications proposed by Weber, von Stein, and Turner. Shapiro, at the American Museum of Natural History, considers these forms as normal growth variants.

From 1932 to 1958, Caldwell, Moloy, D'Esopo and Steer have studied pelvic forms roentgenologically in over 8,000 cases. In not more than an estimated 2 per cent has a recognized cause for the pelvic deformity been found. Rickets accounts for about half of these, or 1 per cent of all pelves studied, and the other half (or 1 per cent) is accounted for by a variety of causes. That leaves approximately 98 per cent of all pelves to be considered normal growth variants. These growth variants are probably hereditary, but the effect of abnormal bone metabolism (other than rickets) cannot be ruled out at this time.

This brief review shows the need of a comprehensive classification. If, as noted above, the great majority of all pelves are normal growth variants, it follows that a classification of pelves which is to prove of maximum clinical value and lead to a better understanding of the mechanism of labor should be based on morphology. It should be sufficiently comprehensive to include rare forms as well as common types. It should provide an accurate description of the pelvic canal as well as the inlet and outlet. The terminology devised should give an accurate concept of the size and shape of the pelvis as a whole.

THE PURE TYPES

In 1933, Caldwell and Moloy,[5] in a classic contribution to obstetric knowledge, introduced a morphologic classification of the female pelvis which consisted of four parent or pure types, each demonstrating a characteristic inlet shape with a characteristic mid and lower pelvic morphology. They suggested a new terminology:

1. The gynecoid type (Gr. *gynē*—woman)
2. The android type (Gr. *andēr*—man)
3. The anthropoid type (Gr. *anthropos*—human)
4. The platypelloid type (Gr. *platy*—flat, *pellis*—bowl or pelvis)

Gynecoid Type (Fig. 8)

The gynecoid pelvis has the following characteristics:
1. A round or slightly ovoid inlet shape
2. A wide, well-rounded forepelvis (anterior segment)
3. A well-rounded, spacious posterior segment
4. A sacrosciatic notch of medium size
5. An average sacral inclination and curvature
6. A wide subpubic arch: "Norman" arch effect
7. Straight side walls, wide interspinous and intertuberous diameters
8. Bones ranging from medium to delicate in structure

Android Type (Fig. 9)

The android type is a female pelvis which possesses major masculine characteristics. The classic architectural features as described for the male are shown in this diagram. Many android types, in living women, show more female features than are shown in this example, as for instance a wider subpubic arch, less convergence of the side walls, and a wider retropubic angle. However, to be classified as android, the inlet should present a wedge-shaped appearance.

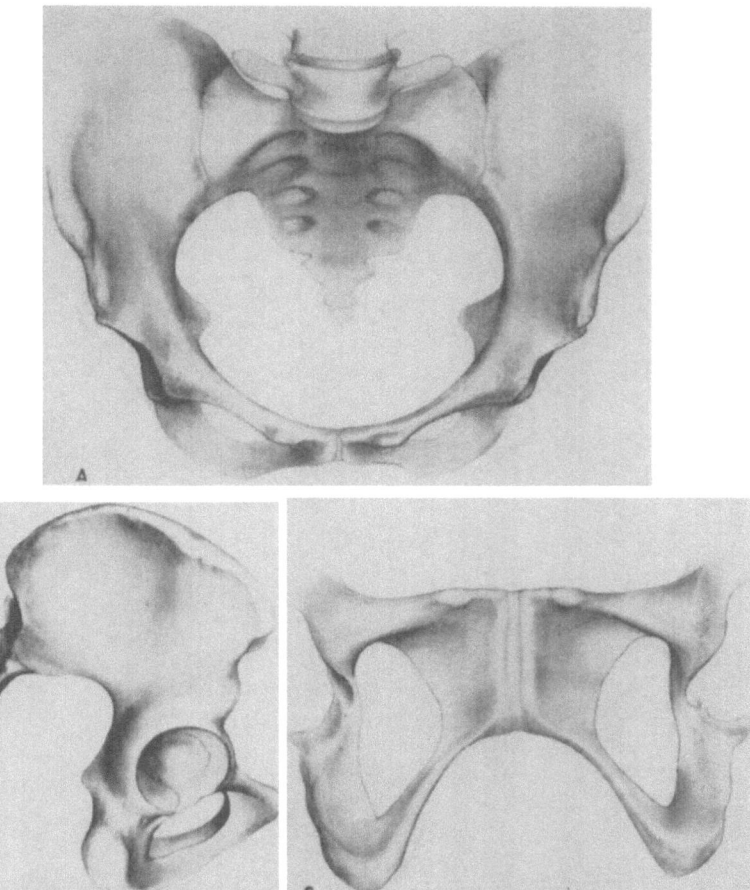

Figure 8. Typical gynecoid pelvis. A, Inlet view: The inlet is nearly round. B, Lateral view: The sacrosciatic notch is of average size. The sacrum has an average inclination. The descending rami of the pubes pass straight down to the tuberosities. C, Subpubic arch view: The arch is spacious and well curved. The side walls are straight.

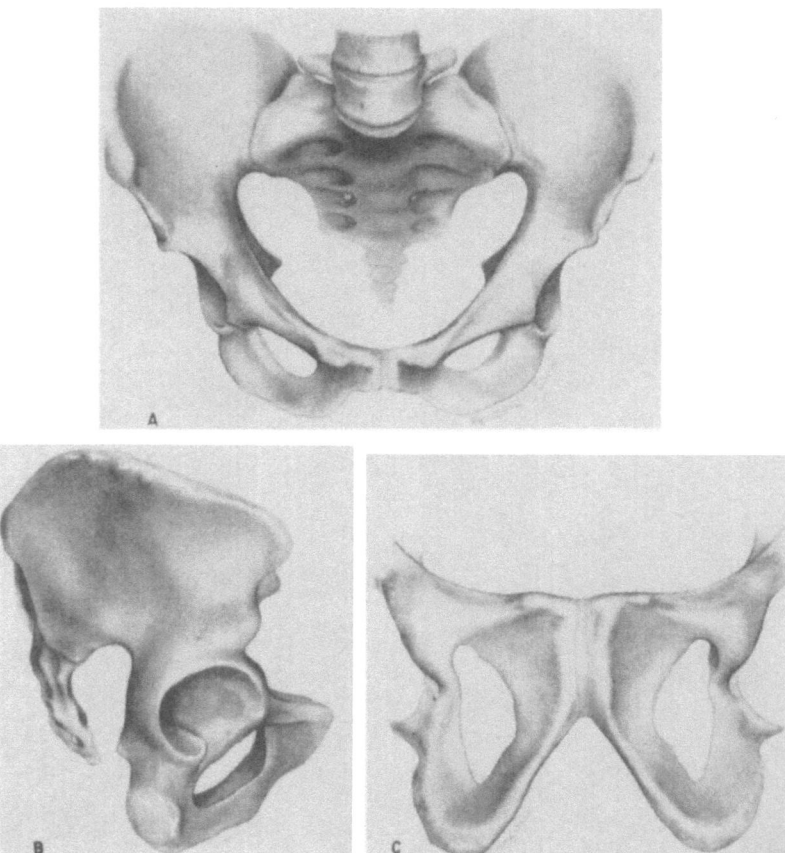

Figure 9. Typical android pelvis. A, Inlet view: The inlet is more triangular than round. The iliopectineal lines are nearly straight, making the forepelvis narrow. The widest transverse diameter is close to the sacrum. B, Lateral view: The sacrosciatic notch is narrow. The sacrum has a forward inclination. The descending rami of the pubes incline backward to the tuberosities. C, Subpubic arch view: The arch is narrow. The descending rami arise from the bottom of the bodies of the pubes and are straight rather than curved. The side walls tend to converge.

The following is a list of android characteristics:

1. Inlet wedge-shaped
2. A narrow retropubic angle (anterior segment)
3. A flat wide posterior segment
4. A narrow sacrosciatic notch
5. A forward sacral inclination
6. A narrow wedge-shaped "Gothic" subpubic arch
7. Converging side walls, narrow interspinous and inter-tuberous diameters
8. Bones ranging from medium to heavy in structure

Anthropoid Type (Fig. 10)

The **inlet has a long oval appearance.** The anteroposterior diameter is longer than in the gynecoid type and the widest transverse diameter is narrower. The posterior segment of the inlet is long and narrow. This shape is caused in part by the **narrow transverse diameter.** The free edge of the first sacral vertebra curves in a manner which further emphasizes the long narrow appearance. The width of the sacrum is reduced in typical examples. The sacrosciatic notch is very wide, greater than in the typical gynecoid type. The sagittal diameter of the posterior segment is long.

The anterior segment is long and narrow, due to a long anterior sagittal diameter, a narrow transverse diameter, and a narrow retropubic angle. In typical examples, however, the iliopectineal lines, deviating from the symphysis, demonstrate a female curvature, giving a rounded effect to the forepelvis. The lateral view reveals the very wide female sacrosciatic notch and backward sacrum. The sacrum, in typical anthropoid types, is long and narrow and often demonstrates the presence of **six sacral vertebrae.** Some anthropoid types show straight side walls and a subpubic arch of moderate size. Other examples of this same type may have converging side walls, with a narrow interspinous and intertuberous diameter and a narrow

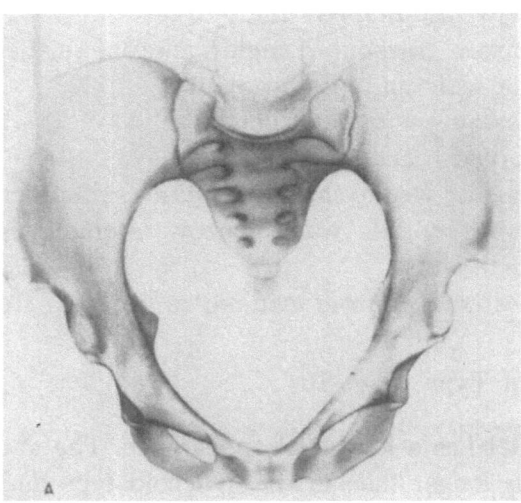

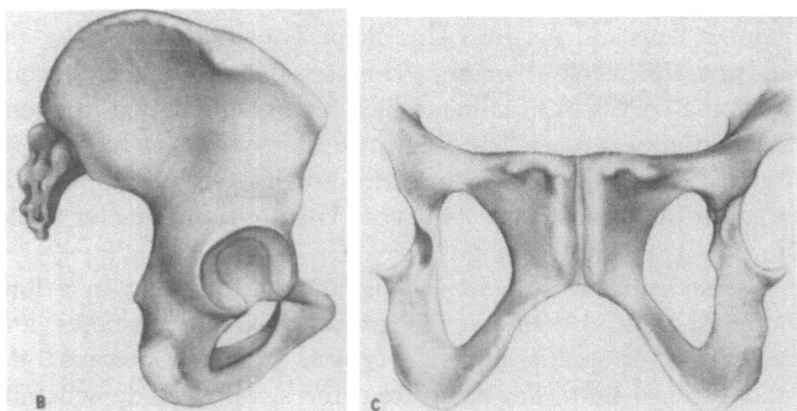

Figure 10. Typical anthropoid pelvis. A, Inlet View: The inlet is long and narrow. The iliopectineal lines are not well curved, so that the forepelvis is narrowed. B, Lateral View: The sacrosciatic notch is wide. The sacrum has an average inclination. The descending rami of the pubes tend to pass backward slightly. C, Subpubic Arch View: The arch is rounded at the top, but the descending rami are less well curved than in the gynecoid type, so that some narrowing of the arch is produced.

subpubic arch. The following are the characteristics of the anthropoid type:

1. Inlet shape, a long narrow oval
2. Long and narrow, well rounded anterior segment
3. Long, narrow posterior segment
4. Very wide, shallow sacrosciatic notch
5. Long narrow sacrum, average inclination and curvature
6. Slightly narrow subpubic arch
7. Straight side walls, interspinous and intertuberous diameters under average
8. Average to delicate bones

Platypelloid Type (Fig. 11)

The typical platypelloid pelvis, commonly called the *flat type*, presents a well formed, transverse oval appearance at the inlet. The transverse diameter is very wide, and the anteroposterior diameter is below normal in size. The widest transverse diameter intersects the anteroposterior diameter closer to its midpoint than in any other type. The sacrosciatic notch, as viewed from the lateral aspect, appears narrow due to the great width of the pelvis. However, if the sacrosciatic notch is studied from an oblique angle, the shape and size approach the gynecoid type.

The side walls are usually straight and the subpubic arch is very wide. Converging side walls have been observed in flat types, occasionally associated with a narrow subpubic arch, but owing to the great width of the inlet, the interspinous and intertuberous diameters usually reach normal dimensions. The typical flat pelvis is shallow, although in many instances this may be a contrasting effect due to the great width of the true pelvic cavity.

The characteristics of this flat type are as follows:

1. Transverse oval inlet shape
2. Very wide, rounded retropubic angle

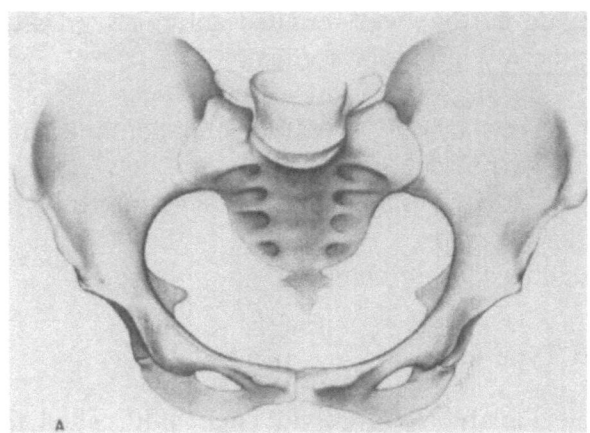

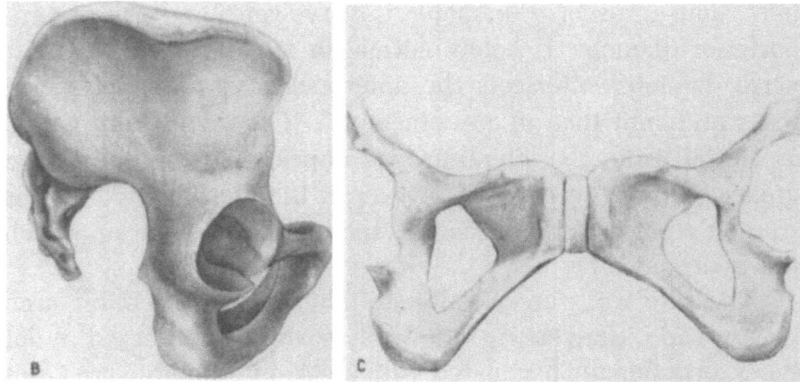

Figure 11. Typical platypelloid (or flat) type. A, Inlet view: The inlet is a wide, transverse oval. B, Lateral view: The sacrosciatic notch *appears* narrow, because it passes in a more transverse direction, although it is actually wide. The descending rami are straight. C, Subpubic arch view: The arch is very wide throughout.

3. Very wide, flat posterior segment

4. Narrow sacrosciatic notch

5. Average sacral inclination

6. Very wide subpubic arch

7. Straight side walls, very wide interspinous and intertuberous diameters

8. Bones ranging from medium to delicate in structure

MIXED TYPES

The four classic types, as described, occur less frequently than "mixed" forms. There are at least two varieties of "mixed" pelvic types. In one variety the inlet may conform in shape to one of the pure types while the lower pelvis may show convergence of the side walls, a narrow subpubic arch, a forward lower sacrum or some other equally significant deviation from the normal. The other "mixed" form may differ from the classic shape at the inlet as well as in the lower pelvis.

These mixed forms present a problem in classification which may be solved by several methods.[6] The accompanying diagram illustrates the cycle of change in pelvic form most generally recognized, (Fig. 12). It reveals the blending of shapes from the long oval or anthropoid type through the round or gynecoid to the transverse oval or platypelloid form. In this cycle two mixed forms occur, gynecoid-anthropoid and gynecoid-flat combinations. In pelves with superimposed masculine characters, the same cycle of change may be observed, by the occurrence of android-anthropoid, android-gynecoid, and android-flat combinations.

The classification illustrated in Fig. 12 may be adequate for most practical purposes, but mixed forms have been encountered which cannot be classified by this method. Masculine characteristics are also very common and may be observed in certain combinations other than the four masculine types suggested in the diagram. Experience has shown[7] that the principle of combining the posterior segment of one pure type with

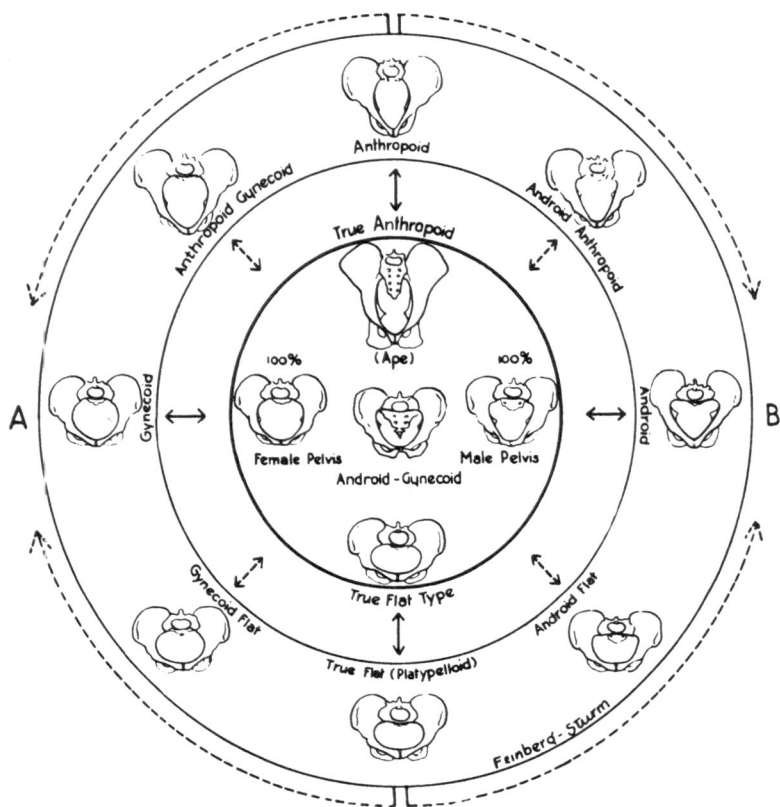

Figure 12. Diagram to show the gradation of change in pelvic form from a longitudinal oval to a transverse oval. Observe the intermediate types between the anthropoid and gynecoid and the gynecoid and flat pure types (to left A). The same cycle of change occurs in android forms; a long narrow wedge-shaped (android-anthropoid), a flat wedge-shaped (android-flat), and blunt heart-shaped form (android-gynecoid) (to right B).

the anterior segment of another has resulted in greater accuracy in the classification of all the morphologic types. The complete classification is outlined below, but more detailed description is necessary to understand the principle of combining anterior and posterior segments.

Each pure type shows a characteristic shape to the anterior and posterior segments at the inlet and also at the mid and lower pelvis (Figs. 8, 9, 10, 11, 13). In the classification of mixed types, the first term indicates the shape of the posterior segment, and the second term the shape of the anterior segment. Theoretically at least, the posterior segment of any one of the four parent types may be combined with the anterior segment of the other three parent types (Figs. 13 & 14). For example, the gynecoid posterior pelvis, when associated with the anterior segment of the anthropoid, android, or flat parent type, results in the "gynecoid-anthropoid," "gynecoid-android," and "gynecoid-flat" type.

The **anthropoid posterior segment** combines commonly with only two **parent anterior segments, the gynecoid** and **android,** to form "anthropoid-gynecoid" and "anthropoid-android" types. The third combination in the group ("anthropoid-flat") is purely theoretical. The "anthropoid-android" type may also be called an "anthropoid type with a narrow forepelvis." At the present time, our knowledge of these variations is too incomplete to permit us to assume that a narrow forepelvis necessarily represents a masculine characteristic in all instances. For example, the term "gynecoid-android type," described above as a gynecoid mixed type, actually refers to a "gynecoid pelvis with a narrow forepelvis." We have encountered a few examples in which the shape of this narrow forepelvis appears to have a masculine characteristic, but in others the narrow forepelvis does not present a masculine appearance. It may resemble the type of narrow forepelvis commonly found in anthropoid forms. The difference between the narrow forepelvis of anthropoid types and the narrow forepelvis of android types exists in the width of the anterior segment at the widest

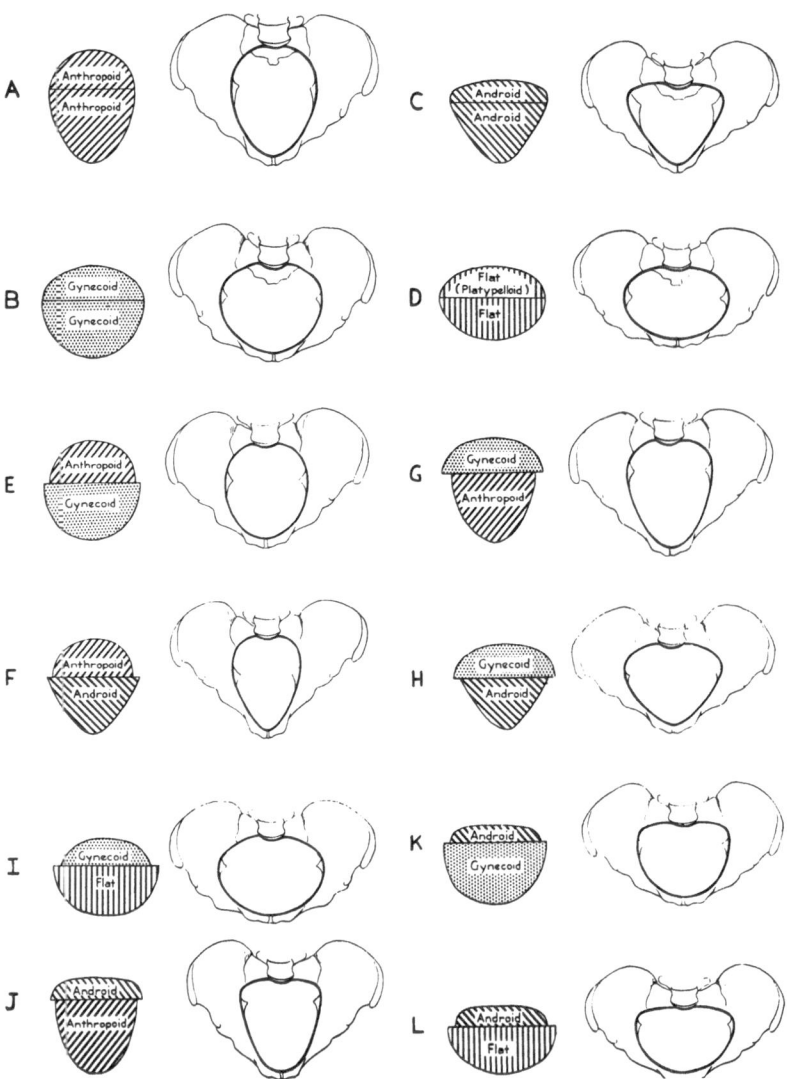

Figure 13.   See opposite page for legend.

transverse diameter and the degree of curvature existing in the iliopectineal lines. The anthropoid anterior segment is long and narrow; while the android anterior segment is wide behind, even though the angle behind the symphysis appears to be narrow. The iliopectineal lines passing backward from the symphysis are straight in the masculine type of forepelvis and more curved in the anthropoid forepelvis even though the forepelvis is narrow in each instance. For classification purposes, however, the android anterior segment when used in combination with a posterior segment indicates that a narrow forepelvis exists at the inlet. Therefore, certain pure anthropoid and gynecoid forms which show slight to marked narrowing in the forepelvis are more correctly classified as "anthropoid-android" or "gynecoid-android" types.

The android posterior segment is frequently found associated with a gynecoid, anthropoid, or flat anterior segment to

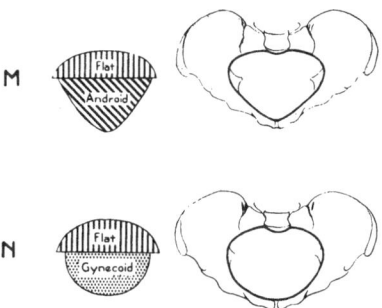

Figure 13. The principle of combining pelvic segments to classify the mixed inlet types. Pure types have a characteristic shape to the anterior and posterior segments (A–D). Mixed forms are classified by the combination of segments. The first term of a combination designates the posterior segment, the second term the anterior segment. A, Pure anthropoid. B, Pure gynecoid. C, Pure android. D, Pure platypelloid (flat). E, Anthropoid-gynecoid (mixed). F, Anthropoid-android (mixed). G, Gynecoid-anthropoid (mixed). H, Gynecoid-android (mixed). I, Gynecoid-flat (mixed). J, Android-anthropoid (mixed). K, Android-gynecoid (mixed). L, Android-flat (mixed). M, Flat-android (mixed). N, Flat-gynecoid (mixed).

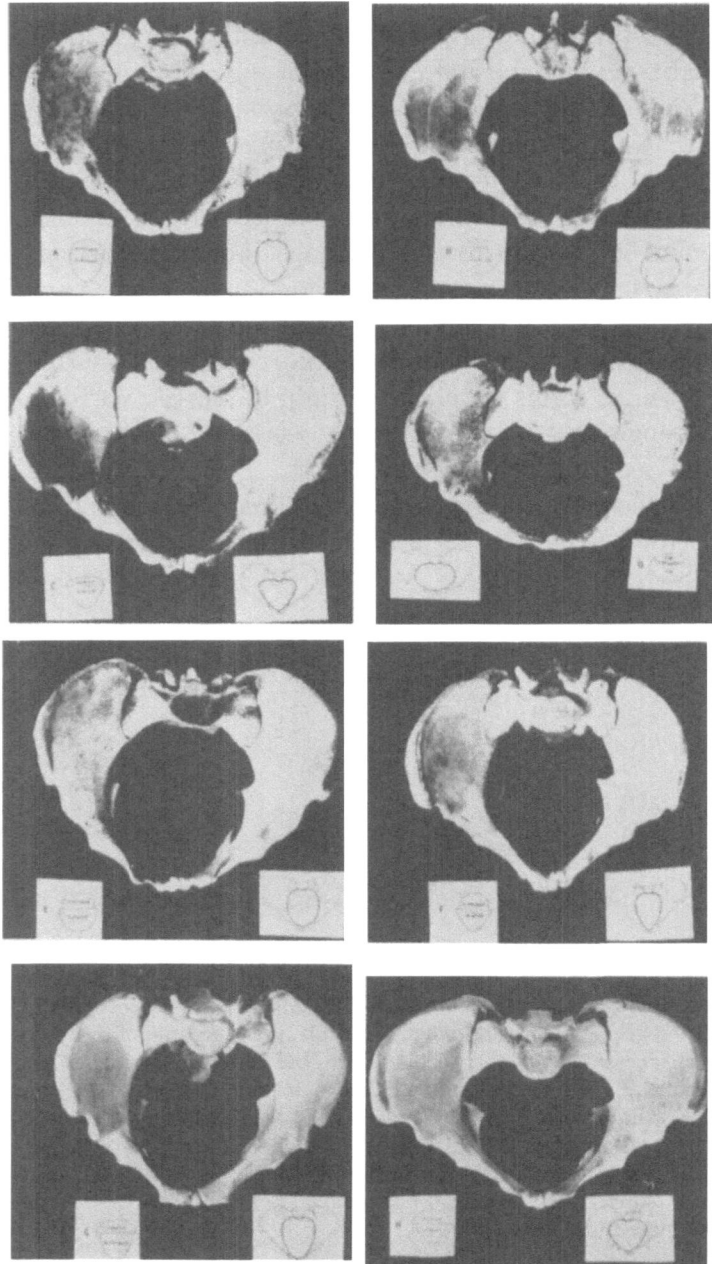

Figure 14. See opposite page for legend.

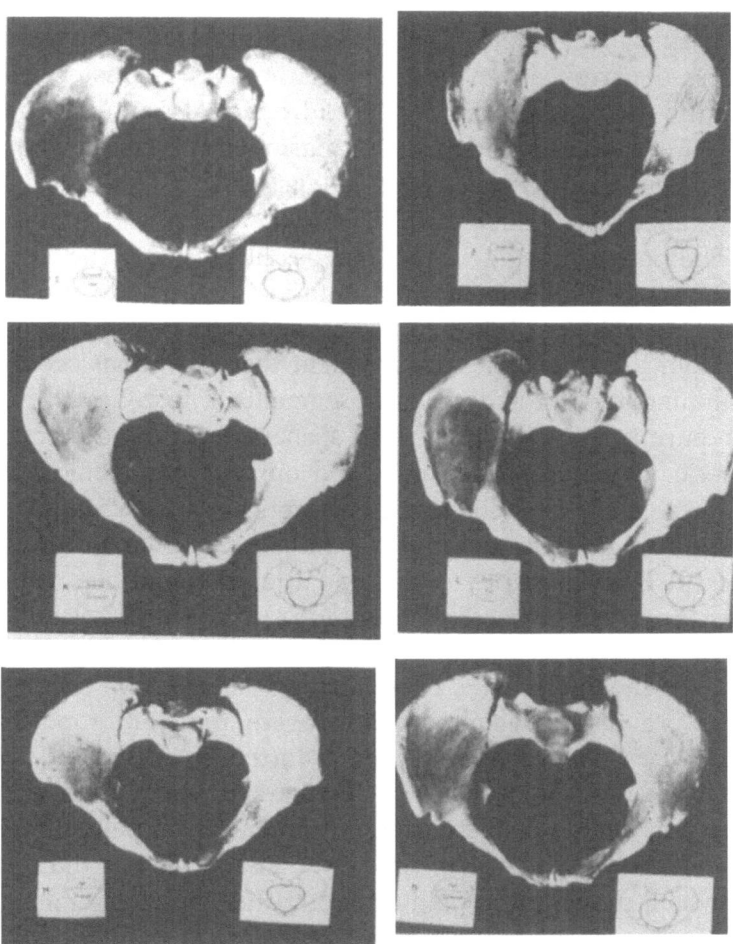

Figure 14. Inlet views of four pure (A–D) and ten intermediate types (E–N) with inserts to show origin of segments and terminology to designate type. The key for the terminology is illustrated in Fig. 13.

produce "android-anthropoid," "android-gynecoid," and "android-flat" forms. It has been pointed out that the term "android," when used as the second term in mixed forms, indicates a narrow forepelvis. Android-anthropoid types likewise possess a narrow forepelvis. The anthropoid character, indicated by the second term, is caused by the long anterior sagittal diameter in association with a narrow transverse diameter. Android-anthropoid types give a long narrow wedge-shaped appearance to the inlet.

The posterior segment of flat types likewise may be associated with gynecoid or android anterior segments to produce "flat-gynecoid" and "flat-android" mixed types.

From this description it is evident that exceptions occur in combining anterior and posterior segments. Theoretically, from four pure types, each possessing a characteristic anterior and posterior segment, sixteen pure and mixed types should arise, but there are exceptions to this theoretical expectation. These exceptions concern the anthropoid-flat and flat-anthropoid types. It is not possible to combine a longitudinal oval with a transverse oval shape. This fact reduces the formal classification to fourteen types. Certain types are occasionally found, however, in which such a combination seems to have occurred. These are pelves which probably were pure anthropoid to begin with, but which have been distorted by rickets. The jutting forward of the promontory and marked lumbo-sacral angle cause a flattening of the posterior segment. Such pelves finally assume a form which is technically "flat-android" at the inlet, but which shows anthropoid characteristics below the inlet.

Another exception applies to a lesser extent to platypelloid-gynecoid combinations and platypelloid-android combinations. In regard to flat-gynecoid combinations it is evident that there is little, if any, difference between the shape of this type and the gynecoid-flat form. The former type is included in the formal classification to denote flat forms which approach more closely to the classic platypelloid form. The gynecoid-flat type approaches more closely to the gynecoid form. The chief difference between these mixed flat forms and the pure platypelloid type is shown in the ratio between the transverse diameter and the true conjugate. In the pure flat form the ratio is as 9 or 10 cm is to 14 cm. In the mixed form the ratio tends to approach the ratio characteristic of the gynecoid type.

The flat-android type is likewise very similar to the android-flat form, but in the latter the widest transverse diameter is closer to the sacrum and in the former the iliopectineal lines are straight, thereby giving less concavity to the wide forepelvis. Convergence of the side walls with a smaller subpubic arch may exist at lower levels. In other words, these flat masculine forms are distinguished by the presence or absence of masculine characters at lower levels in the posterior pelvis or in the forepelvis as well as in the shape of the inlet.

THE MID AND LOWER PELVIS

The Subpubic Arch

The subpubic arch is made up of the symphysis pubis, the inferior aspects of the bodies of the pubes, the descending rami of the pubes, and the medio-inferior aspects of the tuberosities. The typical female arch is of "average" width. There is a shallow curve beneath the pubes, and the rami are well curved, so that a "Norman arch" effect is produced (Fig. 15). This is due to the fact that the descending ramus originates from the *side* of the inferior portion of the body of the pubis. This occurs in gynecoid, anthropoid, and flat forms. The male type of arch has a sharp, narrow angle beneath the pubes, and the rami are straight, so that a "Gothic arch" effect is produced. This is due to the fact that in android pelves the descending ramus originates from the *bottom* of the inferior portion of the body of the pubis.

Variations in the subpubic arch occur in the subpubic angle, the degree of curvature of the descending rami, and the intertuberous distance. In addition, the rami may pass straight

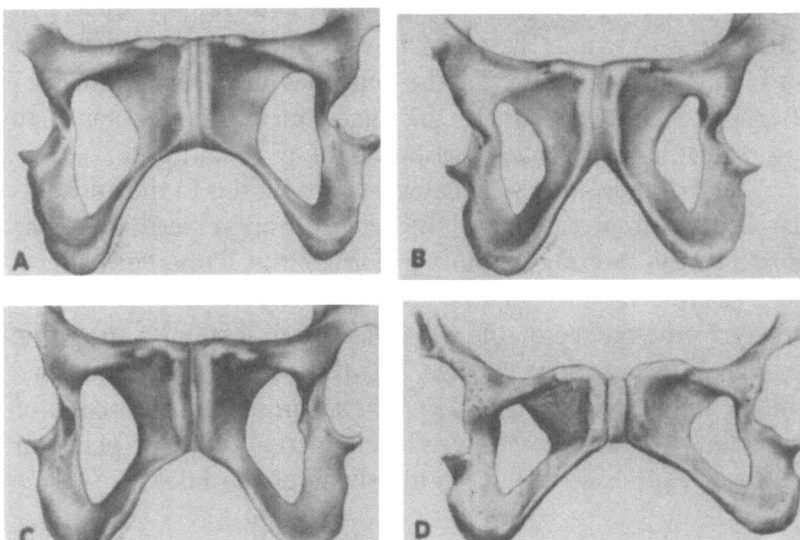

Figure 15. The subpubic arch. A, Average gynecoid form. B, Narrow android form. C, Narrow anthropoid form. D, Wide platypelloid or flat form.

down to the tuberosities (in an anteroposterior dimension) as they usually do, or they may pass backwards to the tuberosities, producing a decrease in the anteroposterior diameters at low levels, as frequently occurs in android pelves. An over-all description of the arch may be made by using the terms "wide," "average," or "narrow."

The Side Walls

The region referred to as the pelvic side walls originates in the upper posterior pelvis, slightly anterior to the upper limits of the sacrosciatic notch, at the point of origin of the widest transverse diameter of the inlet (Fig. 16). From this point, the side walls may be considered a more or less straight line which continues downward and forward to the lower region of the ischial tuberosities at a point which designates the widest diameter of the outlet. A slight convexity, caused by the character of the ischial spine or a slight bulging of the acetabular region, may occur in this line. The degree of divergence, straightness, or convergence of these lines on either side determines the slope of the side walls. Since the lines begin at the point of origin of the widest transverse diameter of the inlet, and terminate at the point of origin of the widest transverse diameter of the outlet, a comparison of the lengths of these two diameters gives a numerical expression of "divergence,"

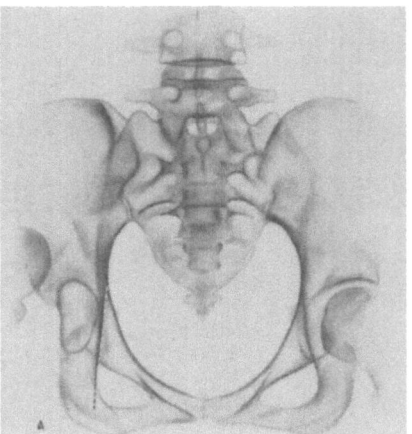

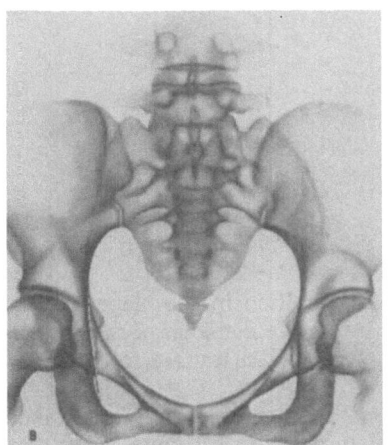
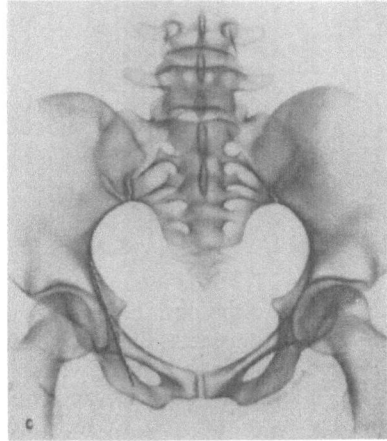

Figure 16. Splay of side walls: A, divergent, B, straight and C, convergent types.

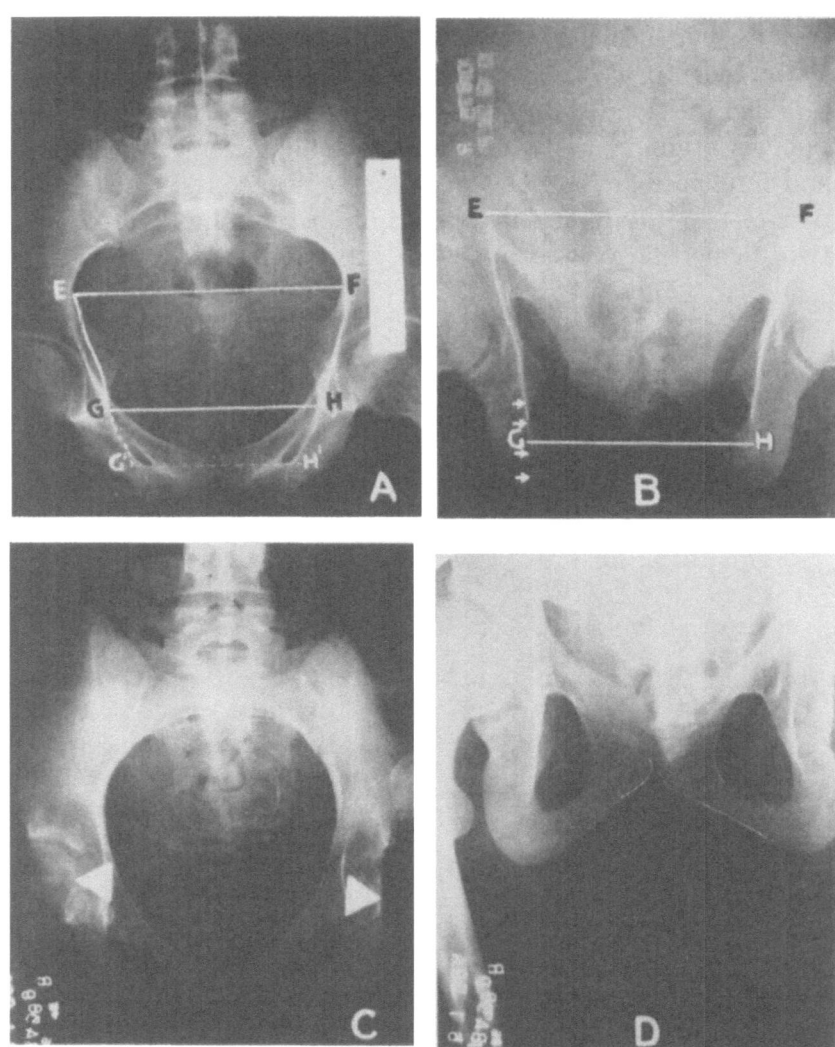

Figure 17. Roentgenograms to show variation in the slope of the side walls and the position of the widest transverse diameter of the outlet. EF—widest transverse diameter of inlet. GH—widest transverse diameter of outlet. EG—slope of side walls.

A, Inlet view. Android-anthropoid with converging side walls and a narrow subpubic arch. Observe how readily the widest diameter of the outlet may be identified (GH). In roentgenologic interpretation any diameter chosen in front of GH gives a smaller and erroneous measure-

"straightness," or "convergence," and these terms may be used for descriptive purposes. Divergent side walls are occasionally found in anthropoid types. These rare but distinct forms have been aptly called "blunderbuss" types by Dr. W. E. Studdiford (Fig. 17, C, D). In the study of roentgenograms, an erroneous point of origin of the intertuberous diameter may be chosen if the line designating the side walls is continued downward beyond the point chosen for the origin of the widest diameter of the outlet (Fig. 17, A, B). A continuation of this line to the edge of the inferior pubic rami does not define the intertuberous diameter but merely a diameter between two points located around the concavity of the lower forepelvis on the pubic rami.

Usually there is a close correlation between the size of the subpubic arch and the degree of divergence, straightness, or convergence of the side walls. But exceptions to this principle occur and it has been found that the presence of a small subpubic arch is no indication of associated side wall convergence in all instances. This interesting observation is illustrated in Fig. 18.

The Ischial Spines

Ischial spines may be "sharp," "average," or "blunt" in shape, and "long," "average," or "short" in length (Fig. 19). The length of the interspinous diameter, therefore, may be

---

ment of the width of the outlet. The diameter GH gives the measurement of a smaller segment of the lower forepelvis.

B, Anteroposterior view of the same pelvis. Observe convergent side walls and narrow subpubic arch. The side wall is straight between base of ischial spine and the bottom of the ischial tuberosity. Above the base of the spine the line EG curves outward and upward toward the inlet to cause a curve to the line EG.

C, Inlet view. Anthropoid type of pelvis with divergent side walls. "Blunderbuss" form. Congenital dislocation of the hip.

D, Anteroposterior view of the same pelvis. Observe divergent side walls and very wide subpubic arch.

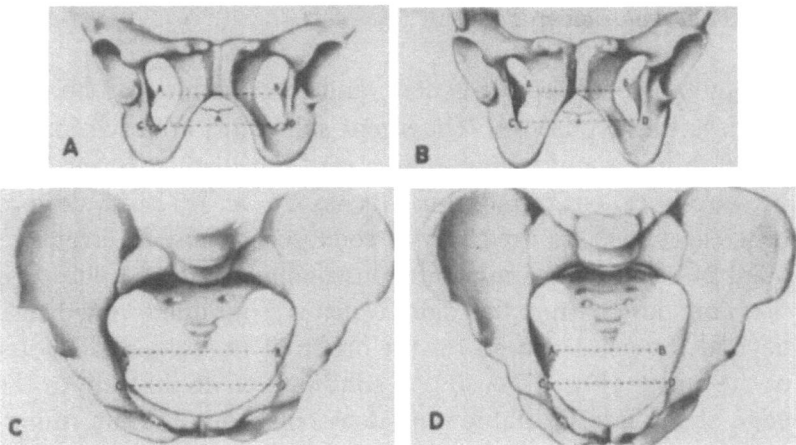

Figure 18. Diagram to show that a narrow subpubic arch alone is no reliable index to the basic pelvic type. It may be associated with either a narrow or a wide intertuberous diameter. AB—interspinous diameter. CD—widest transverse diameter of outlet (intertuberous diameter). A, Narrow subpubic arch A. B, Equally narrowed subpubic arch A. C, Inlet view of A. Wide transverse diameter. Android-flat type, spontaneous delivery in spite of narrow subpubic arch (A). D, Inlet view of B. Convergent side walls with narrow interspinous diameter in an android-anthropoid type. Medium forceps delivery of a small child.

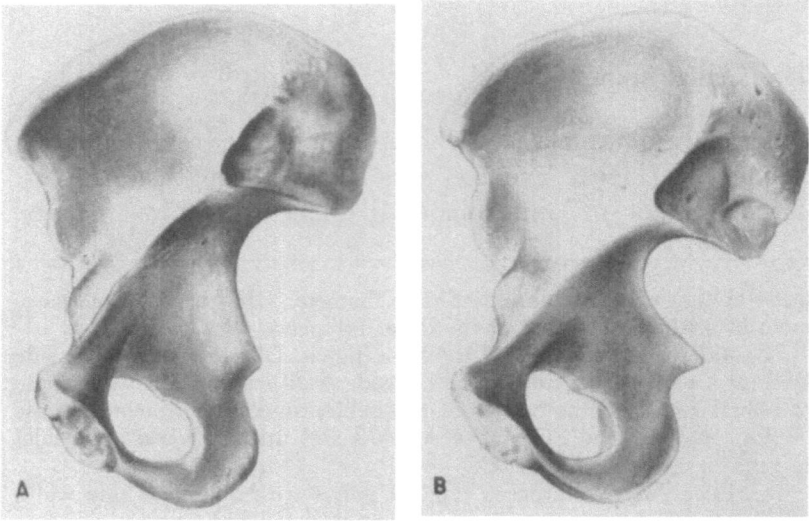

Figure 19. Types of ischial spines. A, Spine on broad base. B, Sharp spine.

dependent upon (1) the slope of the side walls and (2) the length and shape of the ischial spine itself. Long narrow spines may cause a decrease in the length of the interspinous diameter even though the side walls are straight and the widest transverse diameter of the outlet and the subpubic arch is wide. The interspinous diameter is invariably smaller than the widest transverse diameters of the inlet and the outlet.

The Sacrum

Examination of separate sacra will show great diversity in length, width, and number of segments (Fig. 20). The sacrum shows two forms of curvature round its longitudinal axis: the transverse and anteroposterior curvatures. The transverse concavity can be observed through the pelvic inlet (Fig. 21). The anteroposterior concavity is seen to advantage in the lateral roentgenogram, and this curvature determines the inclination of the sacrum and posterior capacity behind and below the ischial spines. The inclination of the upper sacrum may be "backward," "average," or "forward." The curvature may be

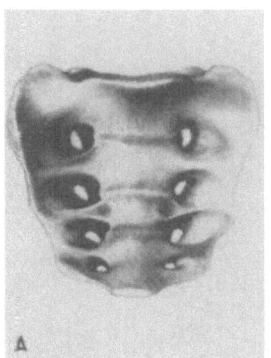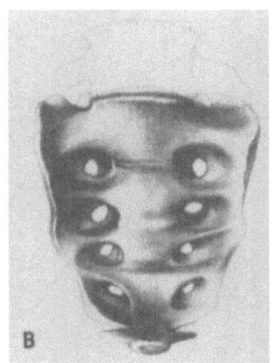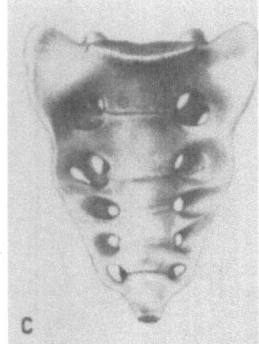

Figure 20. Variations in the sacrum (front view); A, **Short broad female type, five segments.** B, Partial fusion of fifth lumbar vertebra and first coccygeal vertebra. C, Complete fusion of either coocygeal or fifth lumbar vertebra to form a narrow sacrum with 6 segments.

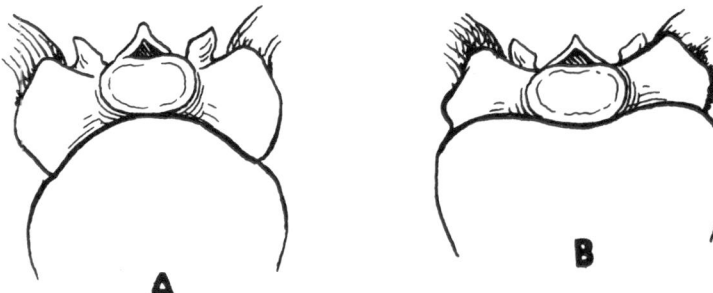

Figure 21.   Transverse sacral concavity. *A,* Markedly concave margin of first sacral segment, common in anthropoid types. *B,* Straight margin to first sacral segment, common in android types.

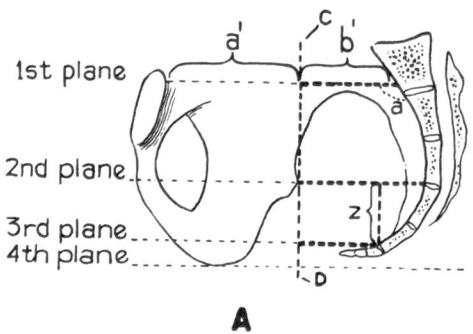

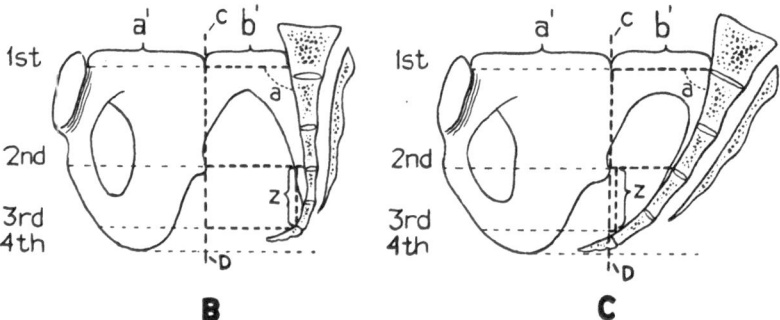

Figure 22.   Longitudinal curvatures and inclinations of the sacrum. A, Backward inclination, marked curvature. B, Average inclination, straight curvature. C, Forward inclination, average curvature.

"marked," "average," or "straight" (Figs. 22 & 23). From the standpoint of lower posterior pelvic capacity, the relationship of the position of the sacral tip or coccyx to the ischial spines has great obstetric significance. The position of the sacral tip may be classified also as "forward," "average," or "backward." The accompanying roentgenograms have been chosen to illustrate common examples of lower sacral variations which may modify posterior pelvic capacity and influence the mechanism of delivery through the pelvic outlet (Fig. 22).

The bore of the pelvis as viewed from the lateral aspect is formed by the slope of the posterior aspects of the symphysis and pubic rami in front and anterior surface of the sacrum behind. Convergent, straight, and divergent types may be recognized (Fig. 23).

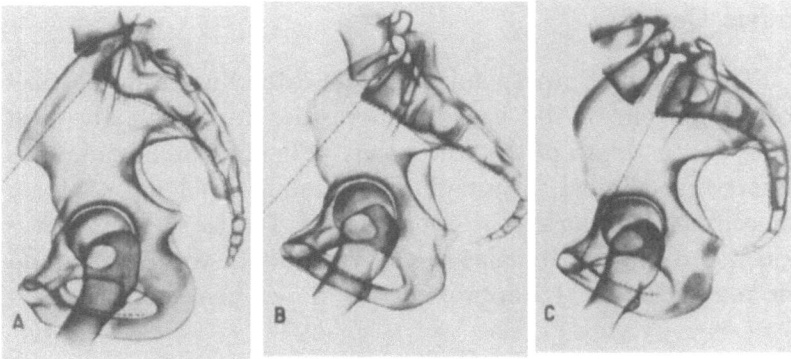

Figure 23. The pelvis from the lateral aspect. Longitudinal curvatures and inclinations of the sacrum to illustrate convergent, straight and divergent lateral bore. A, Convergent lateral bore, forward sacral inclination, average sacral curvature. Plane of first sacral vertebra is above top of the symphysis. B, Straight lateral bore, average sacral inclination, straight sacrum. Plane of first sacral vertebra is above the symphysis. C, Divergent lateral bore, backward inclination, marked sacral curvature, wedge-shaped fifth lumbar vertebra. Plane of first sacral vertebra is below top of the symphysis.

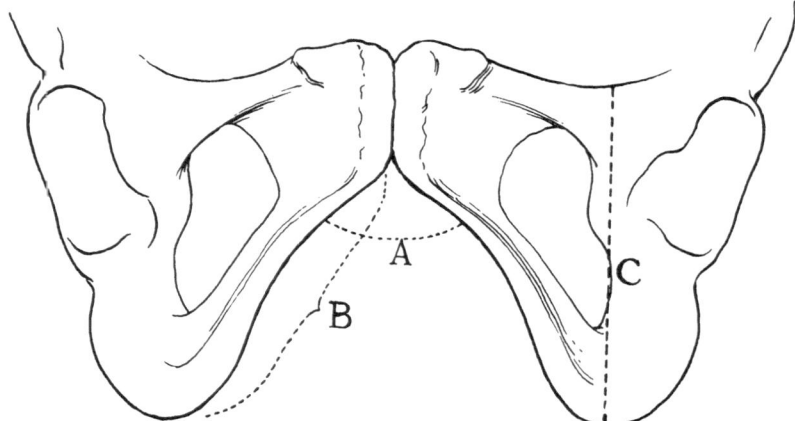

Figure 24. Scheme of analysis of pelvic morphology; subpubic arch
view. A, Size of angle. B, Curvature of rami. C, Depth of pelvis.

Pelvic Depth

The length of a perpendicular line extending from the inlet
to the bottom of the ischial tuberosities represents the best
index of the depth of the true pelvis (Fig. 24). Schumann[8] has
reported a clinical means of determining this length. Moloy
measured this diameter in a number of Todd's skeletal pelves
and noted that for females the average depth was **8.5 cm** and
for males 10 cm. In approximately 6 per cent of the cases,

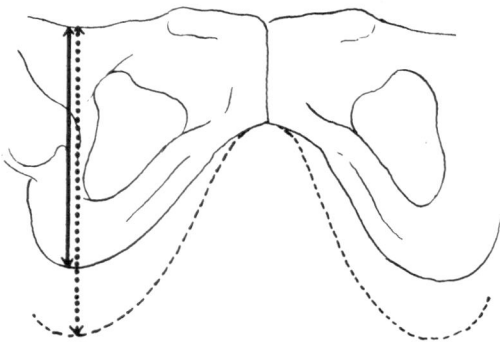

Figure 25. The effect of pelvic depth upon the intertuberous diameter.

female pelves approached the average depth of the male pelvis. The practical significance of increased pelvic depth is obvious (Fig. 25). In large pelves an increase of 1 to 2 cm does not appreciably affect the mechanism of labor, but if the pelvis is below average in size and conforms to characteristic android, anthropoid, or flat types, increased depth in the pelvic cavity becomes important and may help to cause delay in anterior rotation or low arrest of the fetal head.

The Sacrosciatic Notch

The appearance of the sacrosciatic notch as viewed from the lateral aspect shows the presence of masculine or feminine characteristics, and indicates the sagittal capacity existing in the upper posterior pelvis (Fig. 26). The typical female notch is wide and the posterior upper border passes directly backward toward the posterior inferior iliac spine. The masculine type of notch is narrow and the posterior border passes downward to lower levels on the sacrum before terminating at the posterior inferior iliac spine.

It is the size of the apex of the notch which affects posterior pelvic capacity at the inlet. This fact has been pointed out by Derry, Straus, and others through their interest in the sexual

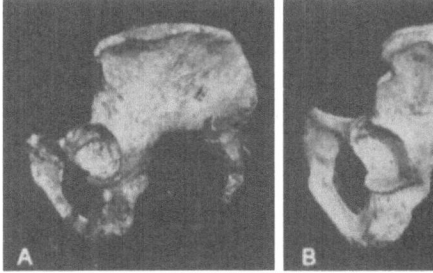

Figure 26. Sexual characteristics of the sacrosciatic notch. A, Female. Wide sacrosciatic notch, backward sacrum. B, Male. Narrow sacrosciatic notch, forward sacrum. (Courtesy of The American Museum of Natural History.)

differences in this region. As Derry's diagram shows (Fig. 6), the apex of the narrow male notch is usually associated with a short iliac segment between the apex and the sacroiliac synchondrosis. This places the widest transverse diameter closer to the sacrum and causes a short posterior sagittal diameter in the typical android posterior segment. The wide female type of notch shows a longer segment of ilium between the apex and the sacroiliac synchondrosis, forming the ample sagittal diameters in the posterior segment of anthropoid and gynecoid pelves. (Compare the size and appearance of the notch in the classic anthropoid, gynecoid, android, and flat types, Figs. 8–11.)

The width of the base of the notch and the sacrosciatic aperture is affected more by the inclination and curvature of the sacrum than by the character of the notch at the apex (see Fig. 26). For this reason, a wrong concept of notch size may be gained if the width of the base of the notch is used as an index. For instance, in certain android types the notch may give the appearance of width because the sacrum has a backward inclination. Actually the apex may be narrow, thereby placing the widest transverse diameter of the inlet closer to the sacrum as in android types. In other instances, the notch may have a narrow masculine appearance from the lateral aspect, yet it may be evident that the notch is ample in size because the sacral surface at this level is far removed from the anterior boundary of the notch. The final classification of notch size into "wide," "average," or "narrow" types may require careful study of the posterior pelvis through the inlet to determine with accuracy the length of the ilium between the widest transverse diameter and the sacroiliac synchondrosis.

Pelvic Size

Measurement of the cardinal pelvic diameters is an essential part of all pelvic studies. These measurements may be obtained by roentgen methods of pelvimetry or by clinical methods. The most significant diameters are the following:

1. The true conjugate diameter or anteroposterior diameter of the inlet. This diameter is situated in the plane of the inlet and extends from the posterior superior aspect of the symphysis to a point below the promontory at the intersection of the ilio-pectineal lines, across the first segment of the sacrum. This diameter may be termed the obstetric conjugate diameter in contrast to the anatomic conjugate diameter which is situated at a higher level and extends from the superior aspect of the symphysis to the sacral promontory. In x-rays, both of these diameters are measured with accuracy by means of a sacral marker placed in the mid sacral region between the gluteal folds for the lateral exposure. As a check on this measurement, these conjugate diameters may be measured from the inlet view by certain roentgen pelvimetry technics.

2. Widest transverse diameter of the inlet.

3. Interspinous diameter.

4. Widest transverse diameter of the outlet.

5. Anterior and posterior sagittal diameters as formed by the scheme suggested in Figure 1. These diameters may be obtained by the method of the sacral marker from the lateral film, but the inspection of the lateral film as illustrated in Figure 22 gives more practical observations than the measured length of individual sagittal diameters.

For well-formed gynecoid types, the length of any one of the cardinal pelvic diameters is a significant expression of its size. While all types may be classified as "large," "average," or "small" in size, it is sometimes difficult to determine pelvic size in anthropoid, android, platypelloid, and certain mixed forms because the recognition of a small diameter does not indicate the amount of compensatory space present in other cardinal diameters. This point is illustrated to advantage in the accompanying diagram (Fig. 27 A), which illustrates that two inlet diameters may fail to give a true concept of the shape of any individual pelvis. In order to record the shape of

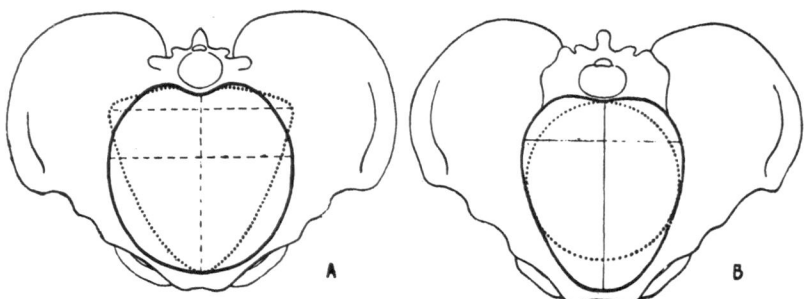

Figure 27. A, Diagram to show that standard inlet diameters may fail to indicate pelvic shape. Both pelves have similar anteroposterior and widest transverse diameters at the inlet, but the inlet shape is different for each. B, Diagram to show difficulty of estimating the obstetric capacity of the pelvis when the shape is abnormal. A circular disk fitted in the inlet gives a good index of inlet size. (Courtesy of Thomas Nelson & Sons and the American Journal of Roentgenology and Radium Therapy.)

the inlet by the use of diameter length, numerous oblique, sagittal, and transverse diameters are necessary. For the same reason, it is difficult to estimate the obstetric capacity of certain pelves with unusual inlet shapes. By the use of a circular disk inserted in the pelvic inlet of an anthropoid type, it may be observed that considerable space exists which may not be available to the fetal head (Fig. 27 B).

Pathologic Pelves

In the 2 per cent of patients at the Sloane Hospital for Women who show definite evidence of pathologic changes in the pelvis, it is interesting to review the forms commonly encountered. It was mentioned previously that rickets accounts for about half of these, or 1 per cent of all pelves studied, and the other half is accounted for by a variety of causes. One excellent example of Naegele's pelvis caused by tuberculous destruction of the sacroiliac joint during childhood has been observed. There sometimes occurs a minor degree of asymmetry in which the affected side appears to demonstrate more masculine features than the unaffected half of the pelvis. This observation was first called to our attention by Dr. W. E. Studdiford. The asymmetry associated with poliomyelitis is different from the minor examples just mentioned. In these cases, the affected side shows marked underdevelopment without materially affecting pelvic capacity. We have several examples of fractured pelves and pelves with separation of the symphysis; the separation in most cases resulted from forceful operative procedures. Several good examples of kyphoscolio-rachitic pelves, as well as two examples of spondylolisthesis, are included in our series.

We have failed to recognize a true infantile type in obstetric patients. No doubt such types exist in females, but we have only observed pelves which may be said to be infantile in young adult males who exhibit evidences of growth abnormalities. We have no example of a true dwarf pelvis in our obstetric material, although a few cases are reported in the literature. Our single example of a dwarf pelvis exists in a 10 year old child who attends a growth clinic in the hospital.

FREQUENCY OF OCCURRENCE OF PELVIC TYPES

In the original edition of this book, the distribution of pelvic types was given in 2 groups of pelves: the skeletal material at Western Reserve, and a group of 215 consecutive primigravid patients at the Sloane Hospital for Women. The pelves were grouped according to the 4 pure types, as nearly as possible, and the result is shown in Table 1. In the intervening years, a careful attempt at typing all patients has been carried out, and the results are shown in Table 2. No attempt at division by race is made. It is apparent that the great majority of patients have gynecoid pelves. The significance of typing becomes apparent when the outcome of labor is correlated with pelvic type, as in Table 3. "Serious arrest" means arrest requiring either mid-forceps or cesarean section for delivery, and the probability of such arrest increases markedly with any departure from the normal gynecoid form.

TABLE 1. DISTRIBUTION OF PELVIC TYPES IN ORIGINAL STUDY

	Western Reserve Material		Sloane Hospital for Women (215 Primigravid women)	
	White %	Negro %	White %	Negro %
Gynecoid type	41.4 —	42.1	44.2 —	47.5
Android type	32.5 —	15.7	22.6 —	8.0
Anthropoid type	23.5 —	40.5	27.6 —	44.5
Platypelloid (flat) type	2.6 —	1.7	5.6 —	0.0
Number of Cases	147	121	177	38

TABLE 2. DISTRIBUTION OF PELVIC TYPES IN MOST RECENT STUDY

Type of Pelves	By Clinical Exam Only		By X-rays		All Cases	
	No.	%	No.	%	No.	%
Gynecoid	7,788	77.9	268	25.4	8,056	73.6
Gynecoid-android	377	3.8	56	5.3	433	3.9
Gynecoid-anthropoid	237	2.4	100	9.5	337	3.1
Gynecoid-flat	54	0.5	25	2.4	94	0.9
Android	256	2.5	53	5.0	309	2.8
Android-gynecoid	172	1.7	68	6.4	240	2.2
Android-anthropoid	29	0.3	36	3.4	65	0.6
Android-flat	3	0.03	17	1.6	20	0.2
Anthropoid	569	5.7	150	14.1	719	6.5
Anthropoid-gynecoid	117	1.2	54	5.1	171	1.5
Anthropoid-android	38	0.4	23	2.2	61	0.6
Flat	115	1.2	59	5.6	174	1.6
Flat-gynecoid	168	1.7	101	9.8	269	2.5
Flat-android	23	0.2	25	2.4	48	4.4
Rachitic	0	0	17	1.6	17	0.2
	9,946		1,052		11,013	

TABLE 3. RELATION OF PELVIC TYPE TO OUTCOME OF LABOR

	Typed by X-Ray		
Type of Pelvis	*Total*	*Cases of Serious Arrest*	*Probability of Serious Arrest (%)*
Gynecoid	268	15	5.6
Gynecoid-android	56	14	25.0
Gynecoid-anthropoid	100	24	24.0
Gynecoid-flat	25	3	12.0
Android	53	14	25.0
Android-gynecoid	68	25	36.8
Android-anthropoid	36	14	38.9
Android-flat	17	7	41.2
Anthropoid	150	43	28.7
Anthropoid-gynecoid	54	5	9.3
Anthropoid-android	23	3	13.0
Flat	59	14	23.7
Flat-gynecoid	101	22	22.0
Flat-android	25	14	56.0
Rachitic	17	3	17.6

Section II

Clinical Examination of the Pelvis

THE ESSENTIAL purpose of clinical examination is to divide pelves into two large groups, the clinically "adequate" and the "inadequate or suspect" forms. The former or "adequate" group includes large examples of the pure and mixed morphologic types which should be considered clinically as "normal" pelves. The "inadequate or suspect" pelvis indicates the presence of deviation from the normal in one or both pelvic segments. It is necessary for record purposes to describe what is meant by a clinically "adequate" or "inadequate" pelvis by the use of a suitable terminology. The following outline has been arranged to serve this purpose. This outline is too comprehensive for use in hospital charts. A condensed form should retain the descriptive terms which are used to describe pelvic morphology for the roentgenologic report.

A. 1. Height   2. Weight   3. Age   4. Race
B. Skeletal status:
    1. Shoulders .... symmetrical-asymmetrical
    2. Thoracic and lumbar spine .... symmetrical-asymmetrical
    3. Michaëlis' rhomboid .... symmetrical-asymmetrical
    4. Lower extremities
C. Symphysis and perineum (patient in lithotomy position):
    1. Perpendicular to horizontal (characteristic of anthropoid types)
    2. Obtuse to horizontal (characteristic of android types)
D. Subpubic arch:
    1. Narrow
    2. Average   Terms such as "slightly narrow," "under average" or "adequate" may be used.
    3. Wide

47

E. Splay of side walls of pelvis:
    1. Convergent
    2. Straight
    3. Divergent
F. Ischial spines:
    1. Not prominent
    2. Average
    3. Prominent or sharp
G. Interspinous diameter:
    1. Narrow
    2. Average
    3. Wide
H. Intertuberous or widest transverse diameter of outlet:
    1. Narrow
    2. Average
    3. Wide
    4. Clinical measurement
I. Sacral tip and coccyx:
    1. Forward
    2. Average
    3. Backward
    4. Length of sagittal diameter at that level
J. Lower sacrum with respect to level of ischial spines:
    1. Low
    2. Average
    3. High
K. Length of sacrospinous ligament:
    1. Short
    2. Average
    3. Long
L. Sacral curvature (longitudinal):
    1. Average
    2. Straight
    3. Marked
M. Retropubic angle:
    1. Narrow
    2. Average
    3. Wide
N. Diagonal conjugate diameter-length (in centimeters)
O. Probable clinical type:
    1. Anthropoid
    2. Gynecoid
    3. Android
    4. Platypelloid
    5. Mixed

P. Pelvic size by clinical estimation:
    1. Small
    2. Average
    3. Large
Q. Obstetrical capacity:
    1. Adequate
    2. Inadequate
    3. Borderline
R. Brief written summary of inlet type and lower pelvic variations
S. Prognosis and indications

TECHNIC OF EXAMINATION

The clinical examination of the pelvis should be conducted in a routine manner, beginning with the subpubic arch and proceeding toward the pelvic inlet until the diagonal conjugate diameter has been measured.

Pelves with converging side walls, a narrow subpubic arch, and a narrow interspinous and intertuberous diameter restrict lateral movement of the examining fingers (Fig. 28). The pres-

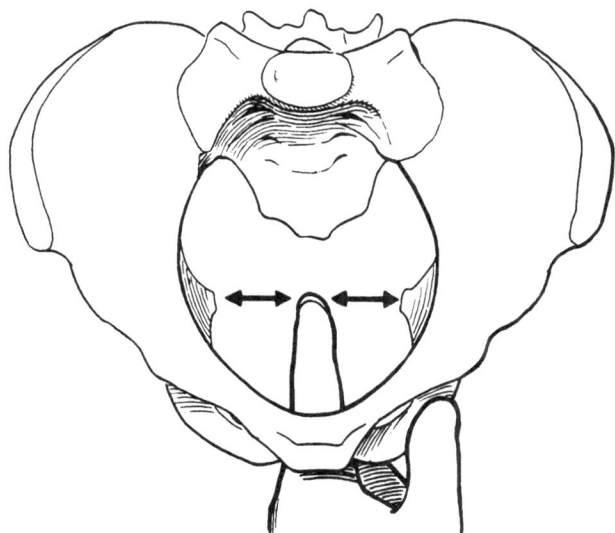

Figure 28. Restriction in lateral motion of fingers in transversely narrowed pelves.

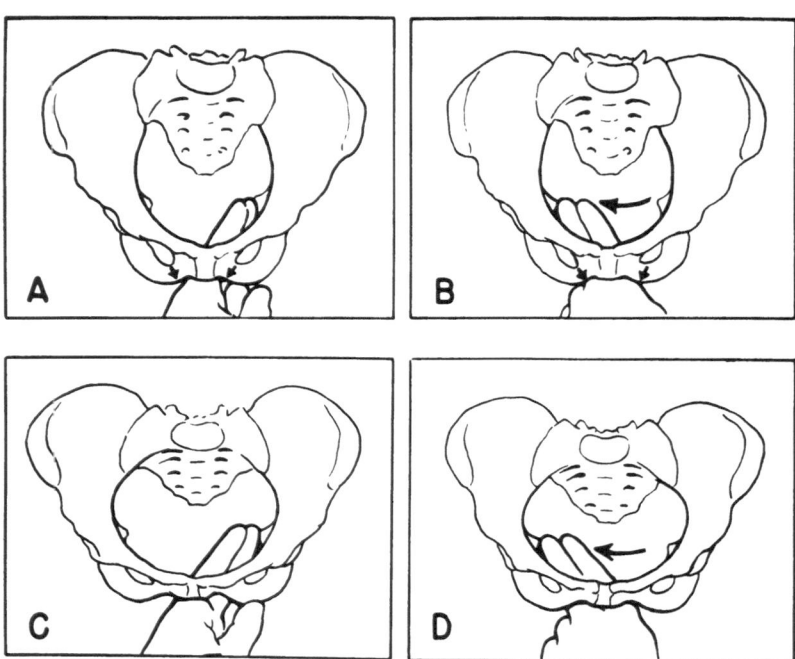

Figure 29.   Estimation of subpubic arch and interspinous diameter by act of pronation. A, B, Anthropoid type with transversely narrowed diameters in mid and lower pelvis. C, D, Gynecoid or flat type with wide transverse diameters in mid and lower pelvis.

sure of the adjacent pelvic soft parts contributes to this sense of restriction. For examination of the interspinous diameter and to a lesser extent for appraisal of the size of the subpubic arch the examining fingers should be maintained in alignment with the long axis of the forearm. The ischial spine on one side is located (Fig. 29). By an act of pronation the examining fingers pass to the opposite spine following the conformation of the pelvic soft parts and *maintaining alignment with the axis of the forearm.* The maneuver is repeated several times. A narrow subpubic arch is evident from the resistance offered to this act of pronation and the examining fingers are displaced downward away from the symphysis (Fig. 29, A, B). The resistance offered to this act of pronation by a narrow arch cannot be appreciated if the fingers become flexed during the maneuver. Flat and other adequate pelvic types with a wide subpubic arch give slight if any resistance under the symphysis to the examining fingers passing from one spine to the other during this act of pronation (Fig. 29, C, D). The observations are recorded by the use of the terminology listed in the outline in sections D, E, and G. The physical characteristics of the ischial spines as interpreted by palpation may be classified as "not prominent," "average" or "prominent," or "shallow," "average" or "sharp." Shallow spines may be difficult to palpate and it may be necessary to follow the sacrospinous ligament to its origin at or near the spine.

There are several methods in use for the identification and clinical measurement of the **intertuberous diameter,** as for instance the Thoms caliper, the clenched fist, or direct palpation of the ischial tuberosities with direct measurement of the diameter. Another method is illustrated in Fig. 30, A, B. The examining fingers palpate the side walls of the forepelvis anterior to the ischial spines in the region of the obturator fossa. The thumb of the examining hand identifies the edge of the pubic ramus and palpation with the thumb upward and downward gives the line of deviation of the ramus. The thumb of the opposite hand locates the point of convergence of the

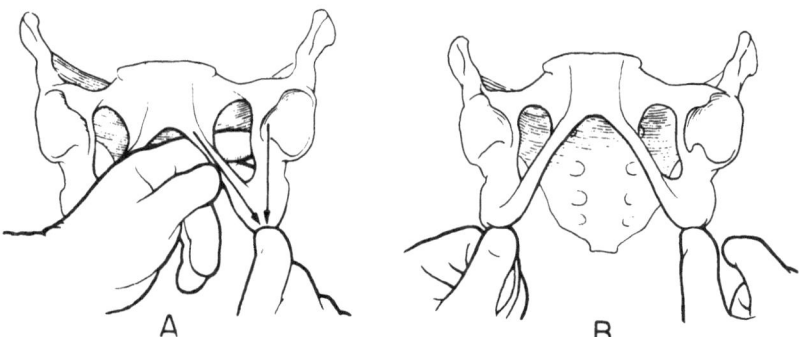

Figure 30. The intertuberous diameter. A, Identification of ischial tuberosity at point of convergence of pubic rami and pelvic side walls. B, Measurement of intertuberous diameter.

two lines at the ischial tuberosity (Fig. 30, A). The intertuberous diameter may be measured in centimeters (Fig.
30, B). Experience has shown, however, that the method illustrated in Fig. 29 is the method of choice for examination of
the subpubic arch, splay of the side walls, and the interspinous
diameter.

The conventional intertuberous diameter and the anterior
and posterior sagittal diameters of the outlet as described in
standard obstetrical texts do not give as good an index of mid
and lower outlet capacity as the interspinous diameter, splay
of the side walls and the size of the subpubic arch. However,
many obstetricians advise the routine measurement of these
conventional outlet diameters.

A clinical method of measuring the "pubotuberous" distance by calipers to give the depth of the true pelvis has been
described by Schuman.[8] This method is comparable to the
index of pelvic depth illustrated in Figs. 24 and 25.

The second important part of the clinical examination of
the mid and lower pelvis concerns the location of the sacral
tip and coccyx with respect to the ischial spines and the posterior aspect of the pubic rami. Bimanual examination as illustrated in Fig. 31 or by the use of the thumb of the examining
hand aids in the identification of the sacrococcygeal joint.
Certain examiners prefer to measure, on the examining fingers,
the distance between the under aspect of the symphysis and
the sacral tip, a diameter which may be called the "diagonal
conjugate of the outlet" (Fig. 32). However, this diameter
does not give the important relationship of the sacral tip to the
level of the ischial spines or the anterior sagittal space in front
of the sacral tip and parallel to the other pelvic planes. The
available space in front of the tip of the sacrum may be estimated by the method illustrated in Fig. 33. The tip of the
sacrum is located by the bimanual method illustrated in Fig.
31 and the thumb of the examining hand identifies the curved
inner aspect of the adjacent section of the pubic ramus. This
distance as measured is a good index of the anterior sagittal

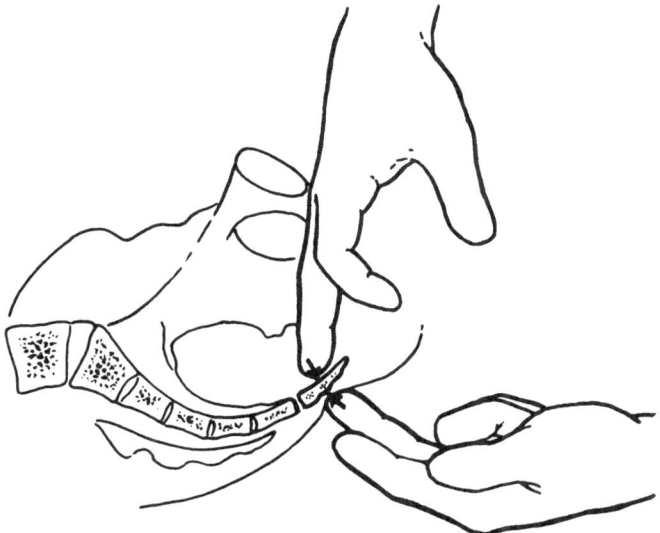

Figure 31. Identification of sacrococcygeal joint.

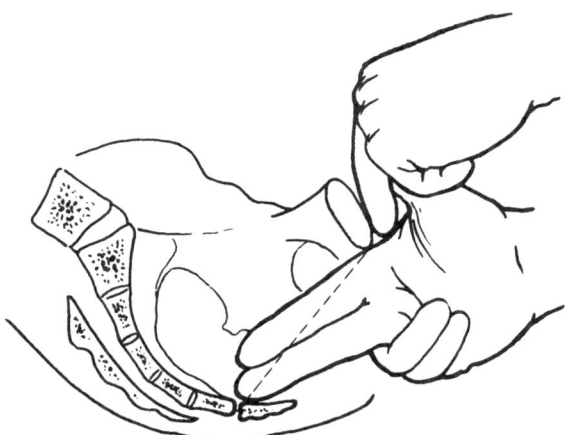

Figure 32. Diagonal conjugate of the outlet.

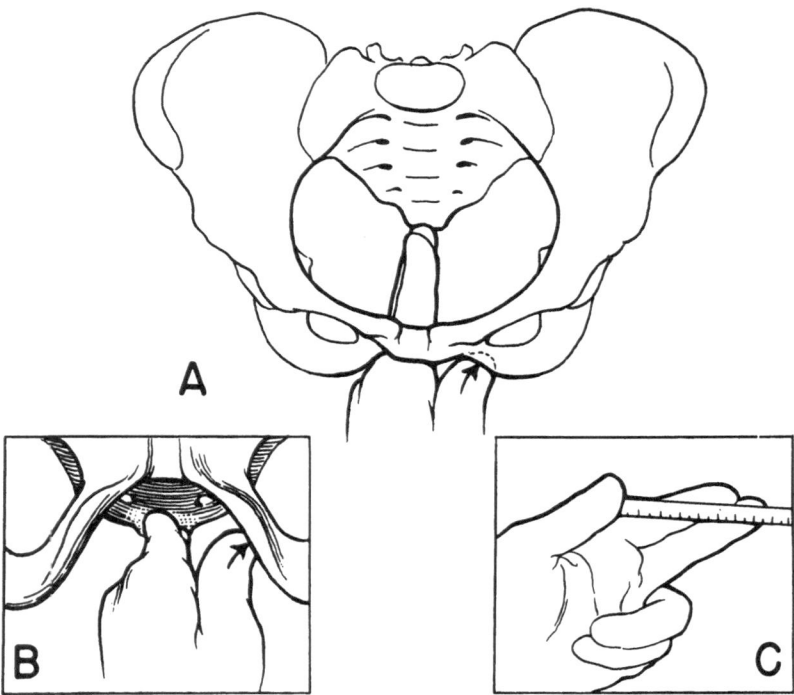

Figure 33.   Estimation of available sagittal space in front of the sacral tip.

space at this level. The distance between the level of the sacral tip and the interspinous diameter may be estimated by placing one finger on the spines and the other on the sacrococcygeal platform in the midline. This maneuver also gives the length of the sacrospinous ligament. The length of the sacrospinous ligament is a good index of the position of the tip of the sacrum and coccyx. A ligament two fingers or less in length is abnormal and suggests the presence of a forward lower sacrum. The average length is approximately three fingers. A very long ligament indicates that the sacral tip is displaced backward.

The method of examination illustrated in Fig. 33 may be employed while performing a rectal examination during labor. In fact, the sacrococcygeal joint is more readily identified by rectal than by vaginal palpation. The index finger locates the sacral tip or coccyx by rectum and the thumb of the examining hand successively palpates the accessible landmarks of the subpubic arch, i.e., the under aspect of the symphysis pubis, pubic rami or ischial tuberosities. It is possible to measure the distance between the sacral tip and the landmark selected by the thumb around the circumference of the subpubic arch. At the same time by palpation of the ischial spines and pelvic side walls it is possible to estimate the degree of adequacy of the interspinous diameter and the size of the subpubic arch. Rectal examination may be used as a routine procedure to estimate outlet capacity at the time of the initial rectal examination during labor. It has considerable educational value as a check upon the routine vaginal examination performed earlier in pregnancy.

The sacrospinous ligaments may be palpated to the ischial spines by rectal examination without discomfort to the patient. However, attempts to estimate the size of the sacrosciatic notch at higher levels in the posterior pelvis by rectal or vaginal examination cause too much discomfort to be used as a routine procedure.

These methods of examination determine the position of the sacral tip in the lower midpelvis and, depending upon the measured length of the diameters as illustrated, the sacral tip may be "forward," "average" or "backward." The recognition of a forward lower sacrum or coccyx is a significant observation. The lower sacrum may extend forward to a marked degree without affecting head mechanism at the outlet provided the sacrum is long and extends forward at a *low* level to the ischial spines. The outlet mechanism is adversely affected if the sacrococcygeal platform is *forward* and *elevated* toward the level of the ischial spines.

Following identification of the position and level of the sacral tip, the sacral curvature and inclination are investigated by palpation of the anterior surface of the sacrum upward toward the promontory. Sacral curvatures are classified by such terms as "average," "marked" or "straight" and the inclination is described as "forward," "average" or "backward." This part

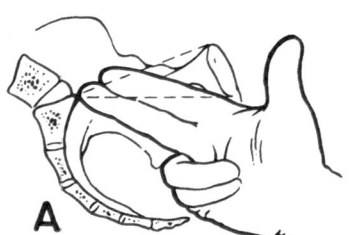 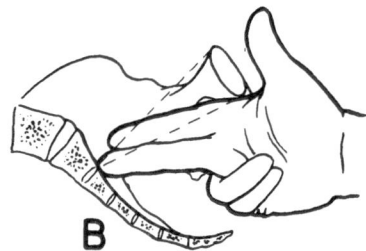

Figure 34. The diagonal conjugate diameter of the inlet. A, When the examining finger definitely reaches the promontory, the true conjugate diameter may be estimated by subtracting 1 to 1.5 cm. from the measured length of the diagonal conjugate diameter. B, If the examining finger fails to reach the promontory, the measured length of the diagonal conjugate diameter may give the length of the anteroposterior diameter of the inlet.

of the examination is carried out during the investigation of the diagonal conjugate diameter.

The third step in the examination is the measurement of the diagonal conjugate diameter with the fingers and forearm in alignment. The method of identification and measurement of the diagonal conjugate is well known to all obstetricians. However, to reach the promontory of the sacrum, especially if it overhangs the posterior aspect of the inlet, the elbow should be lowered to allow the examining fingers to be directed upward at an acute angle toward the upper sacrum (Fig. 34, A). This maneuver is advised as a routine because failure to reach the midpoint of the sacrum may lead the examiner to conclude that the diagonal conjugate diameter is adequate at the inlet. A forward overhanging promontory is commonly associated with a backward sacral inclination or marked sacral concavity. If the examining finger reaches the high level of the promontory of the sacrum, the true conjugate diameter is estimated by subtracting the conventional 1 to 1.5 cm from the measured length of the diagonal conjugate diameter (Fig. 34, A). Except in rare instances, it is difficult to reach the promontory even though restriction exists in the length of the diagonal conjugate diameter and, by chance, the diameter may be measured from a point on the anterior surface of the sacrum below the anatomical promontory. Under these circumstances the measured length of the diagonal conjugate diameter may give the actual anteroposterior diameter of the inlet because the sacral origin of the diameter selected by chance may bear an isosceles triangle relationship to the superior and inferior edge of the symphysis (Fig. 34 B).

Certain obstetricians hold the opinion that a brief written summary of the pelvic deviations is more significant than an attempt to classify the pelvis according to its morphologic type. However, in most instances it is possible to make a clinical diagnosis of the inlet morphology upon the basis of the results obtained from a comprehensive clinical examination. The following outline illustrates how inlet morphology may be inferred from the characteristics of the mid and lower pelvis.

1. In general, the characteristics of the anterior segment of the inlet will correspond with the anterior portion of the lower pelvis. A subpubic arch with a well-rounded apex, curved rami, and space between the tuberosities for the clenched fist, together with straight side walls, will be associated with a well rounded, *gynecoid* anterior segment of the inlet. A narrow subpubic arch, with a narrow angle and straight rami, together with convergent side walls and heavy spines, will be associated with a narrowed, *android* anterior segment of the inlet. A narrow subpubic arch, with a rounded apex and slightly curved rami, together with straight side walls and a narrowed interspinous diameter, will be associated with an *anthropoid* anterior segment of the inlet. A very wide subpubic arch, with straight to divergent side walls and a wide interspinous diameter, will be associated with a *flat* anterior segment of the inlet. It is often possible, by flexing the fingers against the posterior aspect of the pubes and moving them from side to side, to palpate a portion of the anterior segment. When this can be done, confirmation of the impression gained from the lower pelvis can be obtained.

2. The posterior segment of the inlet can not be palpated.

Since this is formed by the ilia and the sacrum, it is possible to type this segment by palpation of the lower pelvis. In most instances, the length of the sacrospinous ligament is an index of the size of the sacrosciatic notch. Thus, a narrow notch will be associated with a sacrospinous ligament two finger breadths in length, or less. Such a notch is *android,* and the posterior inlet will also be android. A ligament of 2½ to 3 finger breadths indicates a *gynecoid* notch, and hence a gynecoid posterior inlet. A ligament greater than 3 finger breadths in length indicates a wide notch. If the ligament passes well backward, and the spines are relatively close together, the notch (and posterior inlet) will be *anthropoid.* If the ligament passes more laterally, and the spines are far apart, the notch (and posterior inlet) will be *flat.*

There are exceptions to this rule in perhaps 10 per cent of patients. These exceptions are due to variations in the sacrum which are independent of the basic pelvic type. The inclination and curvature of the sacrum can be altered by metabolic factors or injury. Errors in the clinical typing of the posterior segment are bound to occur for this reason. It is therefore necessary to palpate as much of the sacrum as possible, to determine whether a marked alteration in the sacrum has occurred.

Since the time of Denman[9] the diagnostic significance of the diagonal conjugate diameter has been emphasized to medical students and obstetrical residents to the extent that obvious deviations from the normal in the accessible mid and lower pelvis continue to be overlooked in the routine ante partum clinical examination. Dr. Vant of Edmonton, Alberta, Canada, in a personal communication has revealed the consequences of this attitude. He has observed that practitioners in his locality refer the patient for hospital care when they find a floating head at term along with restriction in the diagonal conjugate diameter. The presence of convergence of the side walls, a narrow interspinous diameter and narrow subpubic arch or a forward lower sacrum, all may be overlooked especially if engagement takes place at term. He and his colleagues are called in consultation frequently under these circumstances.

The pelvis usually corresponds to the anthropoid type with converging side walls because the **android form** with **convergence** is restricted at the inlet and **engagement** fails to **occur.** Forceps delivery under these circumstances may be hazardous and a stillbirth, a shocked infant, separation of the symphysis, or other serious maternal injuries may occur. Medical students, for these reasons, should be instructed in the recognition of these common lower pelvic variations. This aspect of clinical examination of the pelvis is as important as the measurement of the diagonal conjugate diameter.

Correlation studies have shown that clinical methods of examination can attain a practical degree of accuracy not only in the recognition of deviations from the normal, but in the diagnosis of the morphologic pelvic type. Clinical examination in most instances will assist in the selection of patients for roentgenologic examination at term or in early labor. As a result, the incidence of roentgenologic examination has been reduced in our clinic to approximately 10 per cent.

Section III

Mechanism of Labor

THE FETUS

There are several terms that must be defined to describe the position of the fetus in the uterus before discussing the subject of the mechanism of labor.

Attitude (Fig. 35)

Fetal attitude refers to the relation of the various parts of the fetus to each other. The normal attitude is one of universal

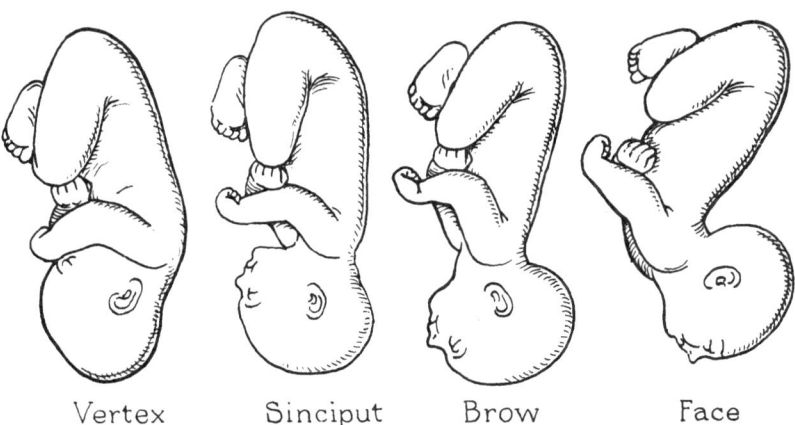

| Vertex | Sinciput | Brow | Face |

Figure 35. Types of cephalic presentation. (Redrawn from A Text Book of Midwifery by R. W. Johnstone, 12th edition.)

61

flexion by which the fetus occupies the least possible space—a reverse squatting position. The fetal spine is arched, and the chin is depressed toward the chest. The limbs are folded in a manner to conform to this state of universal flexion. This attitude is changed by death of the fetus in utero, and an unnatural posture on the part of the limbs, spinal column and head results. In the routine examination of roentgenograms curious deflection attitudes on the part of the fetus may be observed.

Lie

Fetal lie refers to the relationship of the long axis of the fetus to the long axis of the uterus of the mother. There are three types:

1. *Longitudinal lie.* The long axis of the fetus occupies the long axis of the uterus.

2. *Oblique lie.* The long axis of the fetus is oblique to the long axis of the uterus.

3. *Transverse lie.* The long axis of the fetus tends to be at right angles to the long axis of the uterus.

Presentation

Presentation refers to that pole of the fetus which occupies the lower portion of the uterus. With a longitudinal lie two types may occur, cephalic or head presentation, and breech or pelvic presentation.

Cephalic Presentations

With a cephalic or head presentation several types are recognized based upon varying degrees of head flexion (Fig. 35).

1. Normal head or vertex
2. Incomplete flexion or sinciput
3. Brow
4. Face

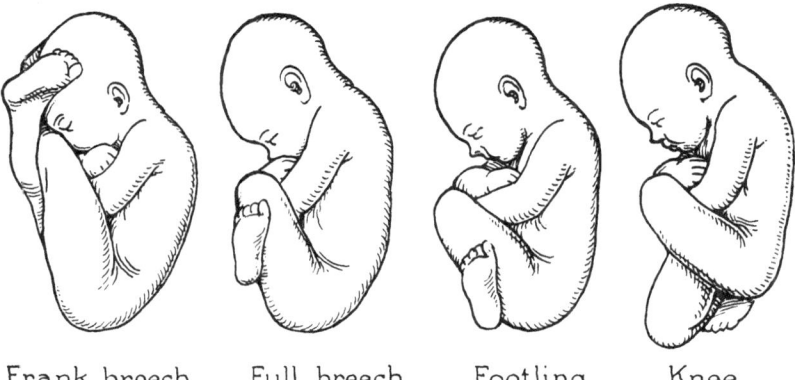

Frank breech   Full breech   Footling   Knee

Figure 36. Types of breech presentation. (Redrawn from A Text Book of Midwifery by R. W. Johnstone, 12th edition.)

Breech Presentations

Breech presentations are classified according to the attitude of the feet (Fig. 36).
1. Frank breech
2. Full breech
3. Footling
4. Knee

Presenting Part

This term refers to the part of the fetus which is felt through the cervix or lower uterine segment on vaginal examination. The terms presentation and presenting part are commonly confused or used incorrectly.

Obstetrical Position

The position of the presentation describes the relationship of the head or breech to the maternal pelvis. For each a denominator is selected and also an anatomical landmark to denote the long axis of the presentation. For head presentations the median sagittal suture serves this purpose and for breech presentations the genital or gluteal fold is used.

Presentation	*Denominator*
Vertex	occiput "O"
Face	chin (mentum) "M"
Breech	sacrum "S"

The long axis of the presentation may occupy any one of the 360 meridians in a circle at the inlet. For simplicity in terminology obstetrical positions are designated by the close proximity of the long axis of the presentation to the sagittal, oblique or transverse planes or axes at the inlet each separated by 45 degrees.

Normal Head Positions

Direct occipitoanterior	O A
Direct occipitoposterior	O P
Right occipitoanterior	R O A
Left occipitoposterior	L O P
Right occipitotransverse	R O T
Left occipitotransverse	L O T
Right occipitoposterior	R O P
Left occipitoanterior	L O A

Face Positions

Direct mentum anterior	M A
Direct mentum posterior	M P
Right mentum anterior	R M A
Left mentum posterior	L M P
Right mentum transverse	R M T
Left mentum transverse	L M T
Right mentum posterior	R M P
Left mentum anterior	L M A

Breech Positions

Direct sacrum anterior	S A
Direct sacrum posterior	S P
Right sacrum anterior	R S A
Left sacrum posterior	L S P
Right sacrum transverse	R S T
Left sacrum transverse	L S T
Right sacrum posterior	R S P
Left sacrum anterior	L S A

The attitude, lie, presentation, and position of the fetus are recognized by abdominal inspection, palpation, auscultation of the fetal heart, and by roentgenologic methods of examination. These methods of examination are described to the student by bedside demonstration or by use of manikins and x-ray viewing cabinets.

Characteristics of the Fetal Head

The fetal head is ovoid in shape with an occipitofrontal diameter of approximately 11.5 cm and a biparietal diameter of 9.5 cm in length. The common head diameters, suture lines and landmarks are illustrated in Fig. 37. The face is solid and the vault is more compressible and moldable. The student is referred to the classic contribution by Holland[10] for details regarding the anatomy of the fetal head, the physical characteristics of molding, and the mechanism of tentorial laceration. Recently Moloy,[11] using roentgenologic methods of examination, demonstrated changes in the base of the skull in extreme examples of molding and described a protective locking mechanism at the lambdoid and coronal suture lines. Head shape is

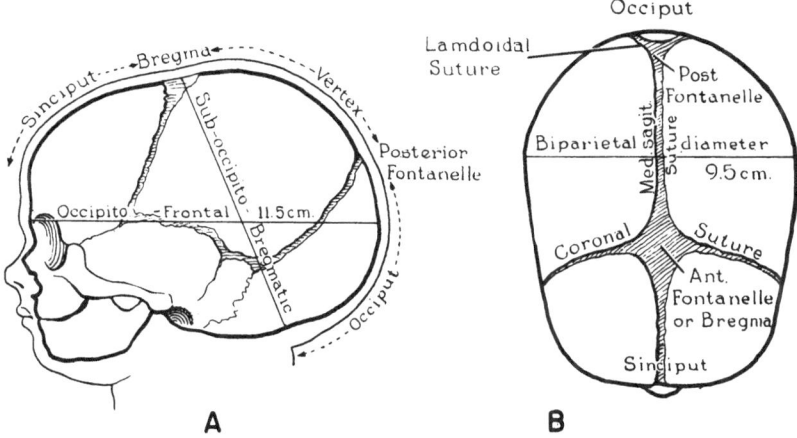

Figure 37. The fetal head. (Redrawn from A Text Book of Midwifery by R. W. Johnstone, 12th edition.)

variable. Round and narrow examples may be encountered. The compressibility of the vault and the ability of the head to mold is also variable due to the degree of calcification and other physical characteristics of the component parts of the cranium. Hard heads mold with difficulty and may or may not indicate post-maturity. Soft heads demonstrate greater mobility at the suture lines, and the cranial bones are more elastic and moldable.

Factors Which Influence Obstetrical Position

In labor by an act of flexion the shape of the projected silhouette of the head changes from the maximum circumference of a brow presentation to the smaller circular outline of the circumference of the biparietal diameter. During the act of engagement the long axis of the ovoid head adapts or adjusts itself to the longest inlet diameter. Accordingly, oblique anterior and oblique posterior positions are more commonly found in anthropoid types and transverse positions occur in flat forms (Fig. 38). This dictum of engagement need not apply to well formed gynecoid pelves or to large examples of other pure or mixed types. In these large adequate pelves the existing obstetrical position may well be caused by the shape of the uterus, the position of the placenta or other unknown soft part factors.

The influence of pelvic shape upon head position is shown in the following table which correlates head position and pelvic

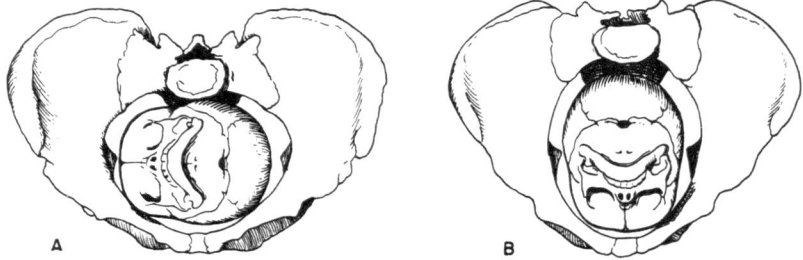

Figure 38. The long axis of the fetal head adjusts to the longest inlet diameter. Transverse positions occur in flat forms (A); and posterior or anterior oblique positions occur in anthropid types (B).

type in a series of 200 cases examined roentgenologically early in labor.

	Gynecoid	Android	Anthropoid	Without Regard to Type
	%	%	%	%
Posterior oblique position	10	20.5	28.5	18.5
Transverse position	69	71.0	37.5	60.0
Anterior oblique position	20	8.5	17.0	16.0
Direct occipito-anterior position	1	0	17.0	5.5

It will be observed that transverse positions in the gynecoid and android types occur in approximately 70 per cent of the cases. An increase in the number of posterior positions with a decrease in the anterior positions occurs in android and anthropoid types. The narrow anterior segment receives the narrow frontal region of the head more readily than the round occiput. As the shape of the pelvis approaches a long oval, the head shows a corresponding tendency to utilize the long inlet diameter. Thus in anthropoid types there is observed a decided increase in the number of posterior and anterior positions with a great decrease in the transversely placed head. In anthropoid and android types the narrow forepelvis favors engagement in the posterior position. A well formed forepelvis receives the occiput and promotes engagement in the anterior oblique position.

THE MECHANISM OF LABOR

The mechanism of labor comprises the various movements by which the head adjusts itself to the pelvis as it descends through the pelvic canal. It may be discussed according to the following outline:

Descent
1. Engagement.
2. Internal rotation.
3. Birth by extension.
4. Restitution.
5. External rotation.

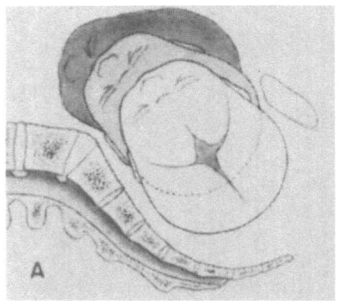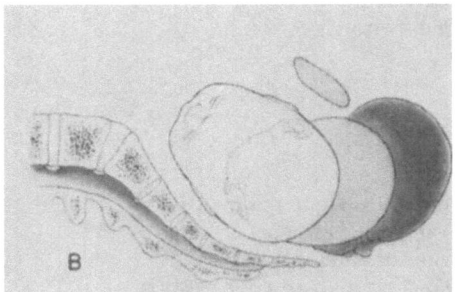

Figure 39. A, Mechanism of engagement and descent to the level for internal rotation. The head engages from a posterior parietal position with the long axis asynclitic to the inlet. The anterior parietal bone descends downward and backward behind the symphysis until the head fits squarely in the pelvic canal. The long axis is now synclitic to the pelvic cavity. B, Mechanism of internal rotation and delivery. The long axis of the head becomes asynclitic again as it moves by anterior lateral flexion downward and forward into the pelvic gutter. Anterior rotation occurs coincident wtih this mechanism.

The first significant aspect of the mechanism occurs during descent to the lower midpelvis. The descent takes place according to the principle illustrated in Fig. 39, A. At the beginning of labor the head usually presents as a transverse position with a slight posterior parietal tendency. The long axis of the head is asynclitic to the plane of the inlet and the axis of the fetal piston is closer to the maternal vertebral column. From this attitude, the anterior parietal bone descends behind the symphysis and the head is carried in a downward and backward direction until it fits squarely in the axis of the birth canal. The long axis of the head is now more synclitic to the pelvic canal than at higher levels. The fetal piston moves forward to assume an angle which is more perpendicular to the inlet. It is a favorable sign to find the fetal piston as perpendicular as possible to the inlet. This mechanism (Fig. 39, A) is described in obstetric texts by the term "leveling." In abnormal pelves, especially the flat type, "leveling" may occur at the inlet before the head engages. At the end of this stage of the mechanism the head has descended to the low midpelvis where internal rotation begins.

The second significant aspect of the mechanism occurs below this level during internal rotation. The head, by an act of anterior lateral flexion (for transverse positions), moves downward and forward in the gutter of the pelvic outlet (Fig. 39, B). The same principle applies for anterior and posterior positions of the occiput. The former moves downward and forward either maintaining flexion or by slight extension. The latter moves downward and forward into the forepelvis, increasing flexion until rotation occurs. Anterior rotation is practically complete when the head has made contact with the lower aspects of the pubic rami. The occiput may come in direct contact with one or the other of the pubic rami at the acme of a contraction. It may be assumed that the flaring pubic rami normally direct the occiput into the subpubic arch. As labor continues the rotation is completed, the occiput engages in the subpubic arch, and birth follows by the act of extension. Restitution and external rotation occur as the shoulders and body of the child pass through the birth canal.

Stereoroentgenograms obtained during labor show that the head may descend through an axis which varies considerably in distance from the symphysis or from the sacrum. This concept is illustrated in Fig. 40. If the head descends through the posterior pelvis, closer to the sacrum than to the symphysis, labor is usually efficient. This axis of descent, of course, is favorable as the head is carried through the most ample diameters of the posterior pelvis. While it seems that descent through the posterior pelvis represents the usual axis of descent, roentgenologic studies show that the mechanism of engagement, as illustrated in Figs. 39, A, B, may take place through the forepelvis close to the symphysis. Although a spontaneous delivery may result, some form of dystocia commonly occurs and the incidence of operative deliveries increases with forepelvic descent.

The explanation for these variations in the axis of descent

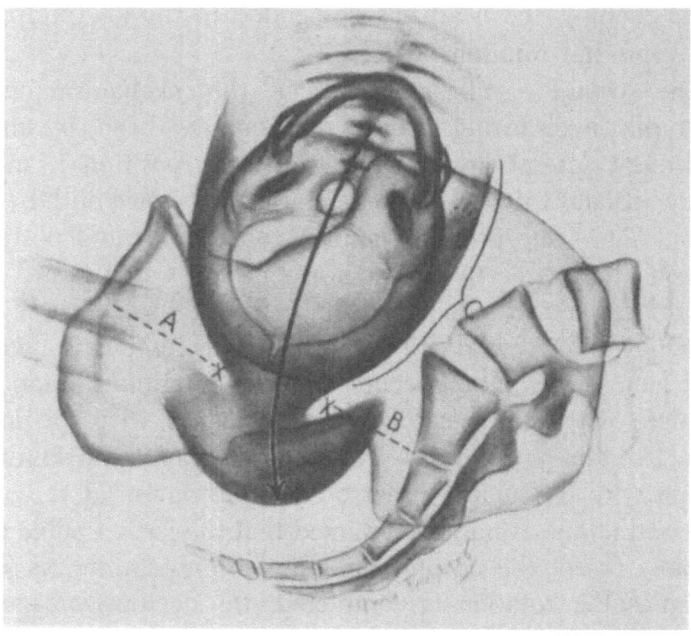

Figure 40. Two important factors in the mechanism of labor diagrammatically illustrated. First, the mechanism of engagement and
descent illustrated in Fig. 39, A, takes place in a downward and backward direction along the axis of the long curved arrow. Second, through
variations in the lengths of AX or BX, this axis of descent may take place
in the forepelvis or through the posterior pelvis.

is not known, but the size and shape of the head, the size and
shape of the pelvis, or the position of the lower uterine segment
and cervix are, no doubt, contributing factors. Barnes in 1860
intimated that the anterior aspect of the lower uterine segment
played a significant role by directing the head downward and
backward. This opinion is confirmed by stereoroentgenograms
and supports the principle of mechanism here described. It is
noteworthy that a definite relationship exists between the position of the cervix and the axis of descent followed by the head.
In descent through the posterior pelvis, the cervix is usually
situated closer to the sacrum than to the symphysis. With
descent through the forepelvis the cervix is usually found in a
more forward position and closer to the symphysis.

RELATIONSHIP OF HEAD POSITION TO PELVIC TYPE AT THE INLET

Three standard obstetric positions of the head are recognized, using the occiput as the denominator: anterior, transverse, and posterior. Intermediate positions which are slightly anterior or posterior to the transverse also occur. As these intermediate positions frequently become transverse positions at lower levels, it seems advisable to place them in the large transverse group. From the study of stereoroentgenograms obtained early in labor, the following data were acquired regarding the frequency of occurrence of these positions of the head with respect to pelvic type.

Engagement in the Gynecoid Type. In the gynecoid group 54 per cent were of the true transverse type. When the posterior and anterior tendencies were included, transverse positions reached the high incidence of 69 per cent. Anterior positions were slightly more than twice as common as posterior positions (21 per cent as against 10 per cent).

Engagement in the Android Type. In the android type, transverse positions of the occiput were noted in 71 per cent of the cases when the anterior and posterior tendencies were included, but the true transverse alone occurred in 54.5 per cent of the cases. Transverse positions are almost three times as common as the combined anterior and posterior positions.

Another effect of the android type upon engagement is the increase in the number of true posterior positions with a corresponding decrease in anterior positions of the occiput (20.5 per cent as against 8.5 per cent). Thus, android types predispose to posterior positions. The marked decrease in anterior oblique positions in android types suggests that the round occiput avoids the narrow forepelvis of android forms.

Engagement in the Anthropoid Type. The number of transverse positions decreased to 37.5 per cent in anthropoid types. Even this may seem an unexpectedly high incidence for this type of pelvis, but it must be recalled that anthropoid mixed forms, possessing ample transverse diameters, were included in this group. In many instances, no doubt, internal rotation occurred before the head had descended to the low midpelvis. The anterior and posterior positions have definitely increased—34 per cent for the anterior and 28.5 per cent for posterior oblique positions. It may be stated in agreement with Fabre and Trillat,[12] Thoms,[13] and others, that the anthropoid type of pelvis predisposes to posterior positions. But anterior positions, particularly the direct occipito-anterior, are also decidedly characteristic of this type of pelvis, a fact not generally appreciated.

In most instances, the head engages and descends in the original position it assumed at the beginning of labor, but it may rotate into the position most favorable for that particular pelvis as engagement occurs (Fig. 41). These observations show that the ovoid head adjusts itself at the inlet to the largest pelvic diameters. Accordingly, transverse positions are common in gynecoid, android, and flat forms, while posterior oblique and anterior oblique positions are more frequent in the long oval or anthropoid type of pelvis.

In the discussion of the mechanism of labor, it was pointed out that descent of the head is usually through the posterior pelvis and occasionally through the forepelvis. Since the shape of the anterior segment and the posterior segment may differ, the obstetric position of the head will be influenced by the shape of the segment through which it descends. This idea is illustrated diagrammatically in Fig. 42. There are, of course, numerous exceptions to this rule because head size and its reaction to the forces of labor by molding and flexion may prevent the expected adaptation. If the long oval shape of the head is substituted for the sphere illustrated in Fig. 42 and the inlet is made to correspond to the shapes of the anterior and posterior segments of the four parent types, the position of the head, characteristically associated with each type, can be explained for each axis of descent (Fig. 43). For gynecoid,

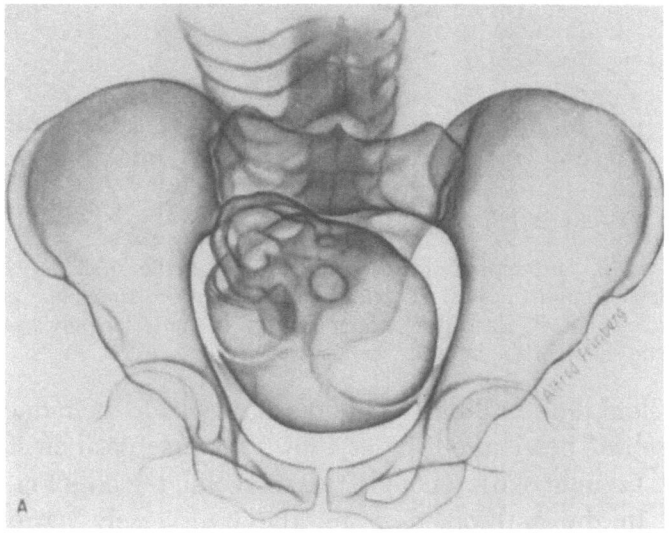

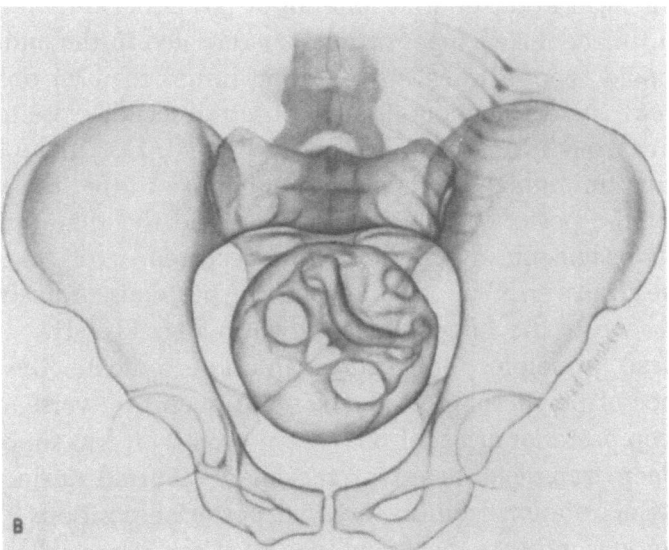

Figure 41. Fetal pelvic adaptation at the inlet. Anthropoid-android type (with a narrow forepelvis). A, At the beginning of labor the vertex presented as an anterior oblique position. B, The head remaining high until membranes ruptured, engaged and rotated in a spiral manner to an oblique posterior position. The round occiput apparently is not so adaptable to the narrow forepelvis as is the narrower frontal aspect of the head.

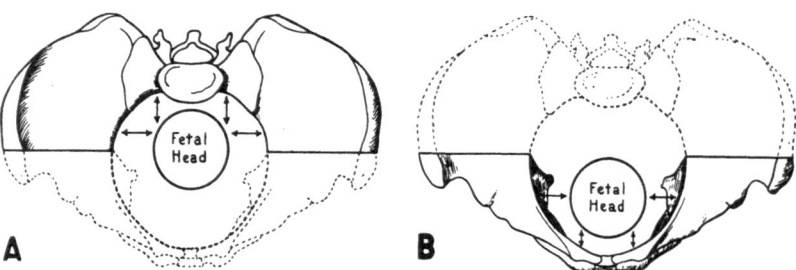

Figure 42. Principles of head adaptation at the inlet. A, Head descending through the posterior pelvis adapts itself to the shape of the posterior segment. B, Head descending through the anterior pelvis adapts itself to the shape of the anterior segment.

platypelloid, and android types, the flat straight boundary of the posterior pelvis predisposes to a transverse position if the head is brought close enough to the sacral region (Fig. 43, A, B). In the anthropoid types, the transversely narrowed inlet, in association with the sacral concavity, most easily admits the head in the oblique anterior or posterior position (Fig. 43, C). In the mixed types of inlet, as revealed in the android-anthropoid type, a transverse position rather than an oblique posterior position may obtain if the head descends close to the sacrum through the posterior pelvis (Fig. 43, D). If the head descends through the forepelvis in this mixed type, the influence of the posterior pelvis is removed and the shape of the anterior segment determines the occurrence of anterior oblique, transverse, or posterior oblique positions. Adjustment of the head to the forepelvis is shown in Fig. 43 E-H.

These principles of head adaptation indicate the importance of pelvic shape in the cause of deep transverse arrest and deep posterior arrest of the head. Formerly it was supposed that deep transverse arrest of the head occurred during the process of rotation from an original posterior position. These observations indicate that transverse positions are usually original positions which have been maintained from higher levels.

In the preceding text an effort has been made to point out the variations in the axis of descent and the role of pelvic shape in determining the obstetric position of the head. These two factors are important in the management of labor and in

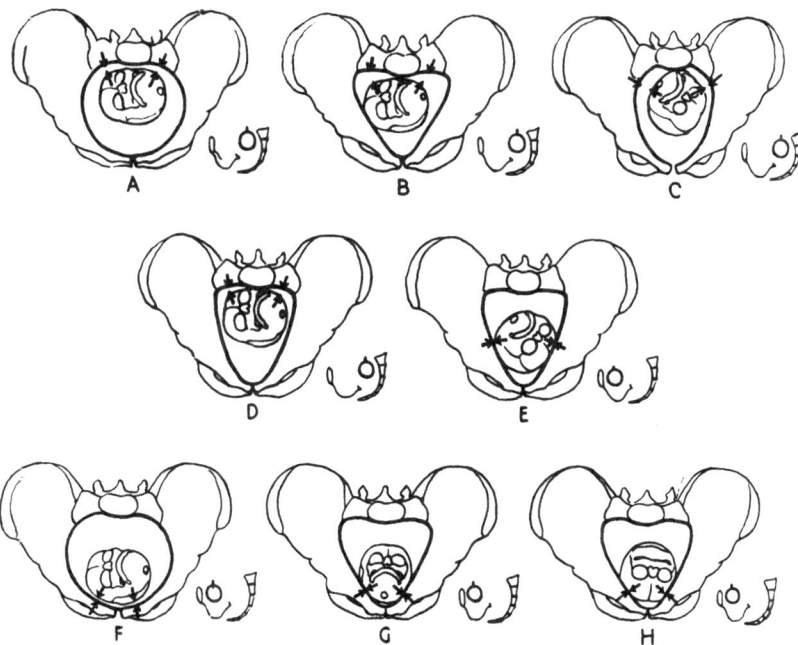

Figure 43. Adaptation of fetal head to pelvic shape for variable axes of descent. A, Transverse position in gynecoid and platypelloid types caused by the shape of the posterior pelvis as the head descends in the axis through the posterior pelvis. B, Adaptation of head to transverse position in the android type for the same reason. C, Adaptation to the occipitoposterior position, or the oblique anterior position, in the anthropoid type for the same reason. D, Adaptation of the head to the transverse position caused by the flat posterior segment in the android-anthropoid type as head descends through axis in posterior pelvis. E, Adaptation of the head to an occipitoposterior position (or anterior position) as the head descends through axis in the forepelvis in the android-anthropoid type. F, Adaptation of the head to a transverse position with descent through the forepelvis in pelves possessing a wide angle at the inlet (retropubic angle). G, Adaptation of the head to an anterior position in a narrow forepelvis when the head descends through the anterior segment. H, Adaptation of the head to a posterior position in a narrow forepelvis when the head descends through the anterior segment.

the treatment of pelvic arrest. For some years the attending and resident staff of the Sloane Hospital for Women have made a definite attempt to apply this information. The result has been a decrease in the incidence of difficult forceps deliveries without a corresponding increase in cesarean section. Forceps operations have also been performed according to better mechanical principles with a decrease in fetal mortality.

Section IV

Significance of Pelvic Shape

In the Treatment of Pelvic Arrest

Midpelvic Arrest

A common method of delivery used in the treatment of midpelvic arrest consists in the cephalic application of forceps (Barton or Kielland forceps) to the transverse position with anterior lateral flexion, descent to the pelvic floor in the same position, and low anterior rotation. Two types of pelves are commonly found associated with this mechanism, the android with straight side walls and the flat type (Fig. 44).

Manual anterior rotation should always be attempted before resorting to more complicated maneuvers. This rotation, however, is not usually successful at the level of the mid or low midpelvis as the pelvis commonly conforms to the flat or android shape which maintains the transverse position to lower levels. In most instances of successful manual anterior rotation, the pelvis showed ample anteroposterior diameters and the delivery was terminated by the cephalic application of forceps to the anterior position. Anterior rotation of the head by forceps from the transverse position is also rarely successful at midpelvis in flat or android forms. The success of this ma-

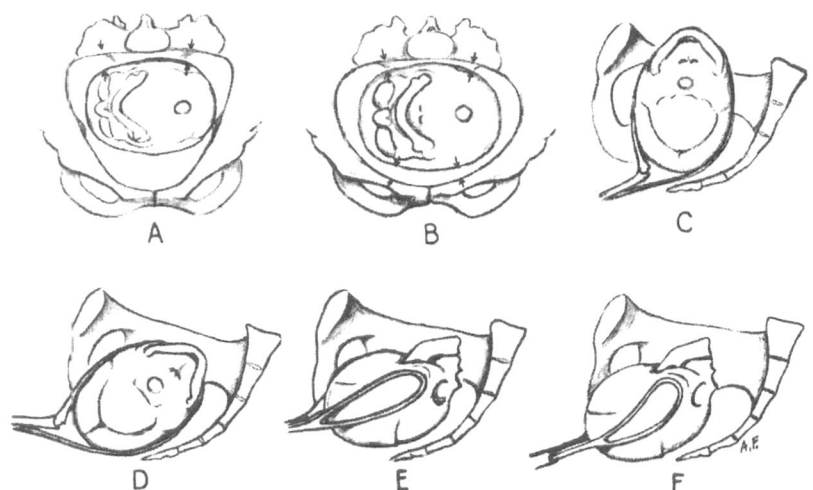

Figure 44.   The mechanism in android types with straight side walls and in the flat type of pelvis. A, Anterior rotation is resisted by the opposing forces between the head and the flat posterior pelvis in certain android types. B, Anterior rotation is resisted by opposing forces between the head and the posterior and anterior walls of the pelvis in flat forms. C, Barton forceps applied to the head. D, Descent with anterior lateral flexion. The head follows the curve of the lower sacrum and coccyx. E, Anterior rotation is effected at a low level on the inner aspects of the pubic rami or under the subpubic arch after the head has been deviated away from the influence of the posterior pelvis. F, Barton forceps are removed and a cephalic application of pelvic curved forceps is made for the low terminal delivery.

neuver, as with manual methods, is dependent upon adequate anteroposterior pelvic diameters or good flexion and molding of the fetal head. The presence of extreme flexion and molding may allow anterior rotation by forceps or by manual methods even though slight degrees of flattening may exist in the pelvis.

The maneuver of anterior spiral rotation with descent is commonly associated with typical android pelves with converging side walls and prominent ischial spines. Although the inlet is not flat, the anteroposterior diameter is usually under average in size and the narrow angle of the forepelvis causes a flat space in the posterior pelvis. Thus transverse arrest at or slightly below the level of the ischial spines is likely to occur.

In the operative delivery, the shape of the upper pelvis acts to maintain this transverse position while the narrow interspinous diameter encourages anterior rotation of the head in an attempt to utilize the compensatory space in the sagittal plane. Further descent in the transverse position will bring the head into contact with the restricted interspinous diameter. Consequently anterior lateral flexion with spiral rotation is the proper mechanism for this type of transverse arrest (Fig. 45).

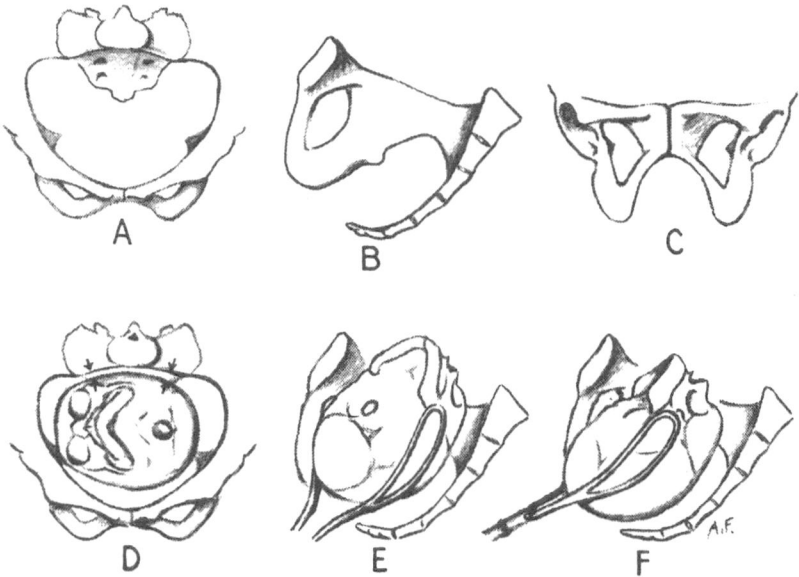

Figure 45. The mechanism of spiral anterior rotation in typical android types. A, Inlet view to show the wedge-shaped inlet with converging wide walls. B, Lateral view to show restricted capacity in the posterior pelvis. C, View of the narrow subpubic arch. D, Transverse arrest of the head in midpelvis. The shape of the posterior pelvis prevents easy anterior rotation of the head. The narrow interspinous diameter with converging side walls below requires anterior rotation in order that the biparietal diameter may descend through the intertuberous diameter and the long axis of the head may adjust itself to the sagittal diameter. E, Pelvic curved forceps effect partial rotation and carry the head away from the posterior pelvis by lateral flexion. With descent, anterior rotation continues as the head moves downward and forward. F, Anterior rotation is now completed with the vertex low on the pelvic floor.

This method must be used with care. Version with breech extraction has occasionally been used to effect delivery in similar cases. It is difficult to study the mechanism in this form because in our series such typical android types are commonly found in the cesarean section group. When spontaneous deliveries have occurred in these extreme android forms, adequate labor has molded the head and overcome bony disproportion. Occasionally, further descent in the transverse position must be carried out, if the posterior pelvis at the inlet prevents anterior rotation. As a result, we have found several examples of android types with convergence of the side walls in which delivery was terminated by the use of Barton forceps. In these cases the Barton forceps served to flex the head laterally into the forepelvis in the transverse position away from the influence of the posterior pelvis. The head descends to a slightly lower level in the transverse position through the widest part of the anterior pelvis in front of the narrow interspinous diameter. Anterior rotation is accomplished at a slightly higher level, but follows the principle illustrated for the flat mechanism in Fig. 44.

The examples shown in Fig. 44 illustrate the head close to the sacrum, descending through the posterior pelvis. Other examples will be found in which the head descends through the forepelvis close to the symphysis. This type of forepelvic arrest may occur in any type of pelvis which presents a flat surface to the lateral aspects of the fetal head. The mechanism of delivery is shown in Fig. 46 with an android-gynecoid type of pelvis. In the upper pelvis the shape of the posterior segment creates a transverse position. If the ischial spines are long and the interspinous diameter is slightly narrowed, the head may descend diagonally downward and forward to pass in front of the ischial spines and utilize the wide intertuberous diameter in the lower forepelvis. The close approximation of the lateral aspects of the head and the well-formed forepelvis helps to maintain a transverse position at this low level. In the delivery, the head should be flexed laterally away from the

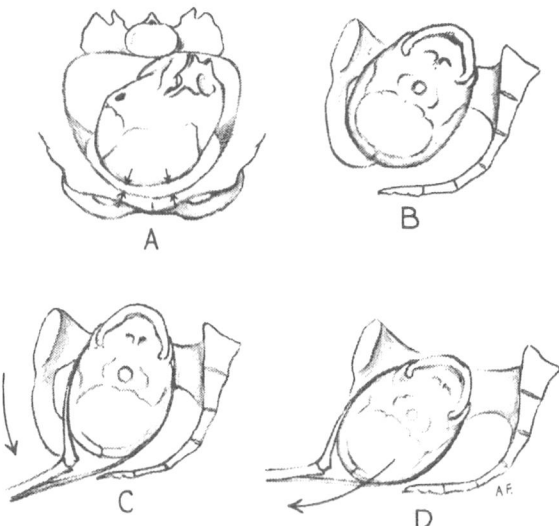

Figure 46. The mechanism with arrest in the forepelvis close to the symphysis and descending pubic rami. A, Arrest in the forepelvis in the transverse position. Anterior rotation is resisted by the flat surface of the forepelvis. (The head may present close to the symphysis in any position.) B, Lateral view with transverse position illustrated. The lateral side of the head tends to be close to the posterior aspects of the symphysis. C, The head is dislodged upward and then slightly downward and backward by manual or instrumental methods. D, By lateral flexion the head descends into the outlet and under the subpubic arch where anterior rotation is carried out.

symphysis before anterior rotation is attempted, thereby avoiding traction against the lower forepelvis.

Low Medium Arrest in the Transverse Position

It is not unusual to have a spontaneous delivery in a flat type of pelvis in which the transverse mechanism has been maintained to a low level. Following an episiotomy, the head rotates anteriorly in the pubic arch. This is an important observation as it shows the transverse mechanism to be physiologic for flat forms and explains the ease of the mechanism used for flat and certain android forms with Barton forceps

(Fig. 44). Manual rotation to the anterior position is usually more successful in arrest at this low level than in midpelvic arrest. The success of manual anterior rotation, even at this low level, depends upon ample anteroposterior space as found in pelves other than the flat type. Occasionally, in flat pelves low arrest may occur with the head in a position slightly anterior to the transverse. One blade of the forceps may succeed in completing the rotation, using the blade as a vectis. Anterior rotation by forceps is also more successful at the low midpelvic than at higher levels. No doubt the success of this maneuver can be attributed also to the presence of good flexion and molding, in association with ample anteroposterior diameters.

Occasionally in low mid arrest of the head in the transverse position, manual and even instrumental methods of rotation fail if the pelvis conforms to the flat or android type with straight side walls. Barton forceps have been found to be very useful in these cases because they maintain the original position of arrest, as illustrated in Fig. 44. These forceps can direct the head backward away from the symphysis, or forward by lateral flexion so that anterior rotation may be accomplished on the inner aspect of the pubic rami or under the subpubic arch.

It is interesting to note that in no instance was low transverse arrest of the head found in any pelvis of the anthropoid or long oval shape. Low transverse arrest in its relationship to the flat pelvis is analogous to the low occipitoposterior arrest of the head in relation to the anthropoid type of pelvis.

Summary of Transverse Arrest of the Head

Transverse arrest of the head is characteristically associated with either a flat or an android type of pelvis. In delivery, this fact must be appreciated and the transverse position maintained to a low level. If convergence of the side walls exists, then anterior spiral rotation is advisable in android types. Success in manual or forceps rotation at the level of arrest usually implies that an ample anteroposterior diameter is present.

The maneuvers employed for delivery of the mid and low mid arrest in the transverse position may be summarized as follows:

1. Manual anterior rotation at level of arrest or at higher levels.
2. Forceps rotation at level of arrest or at higher levels.
3. Anterior spiral rotation with descent.
4. Maintenance of the transverse position to lower levels followed by low rotation.

TREATMENT OF ARREST IN THE POSTERIOR POSITION

Midpelvic Arrest

The occipitoposterior position was found arrested at mid-pelvis in android and flat pelves slightly more frequently than in anthropoid types (Figs. 47, 48). The posterior position occurs in the upper pelvis because the round occiput cannot adjust itself to the narrow forepelvis as readily as the narrower frontal diameters of the fetal head. But this position is not a physiologic position for android and flat forms, because these types favor descent through the lower pelvis in the transverse position. The delivery is accomplished by manual rotation to the transverse position followed by the application of Barton forceps. The head descended with traction and lateral flexion to a lower level where anterior rotation was performed according to the mechanism illustrated for android and flat forms in Fig. 44. The common pelvic type associated with this mechanism was the android form with slight convergence of the side walls and a good sacral concavity (Fig. 47).

In certain flat pelves with a good sacral concavity, arrest may occur in the posterior position (Fig. 48). In these flat types it is obviously desirable to make use of the wide transverse diameter during delivery. Accordingly, the head is rotated manually to the transverse position and the delivery is terminated by the use of Barton forceps, as illustrated in Fig. 44.

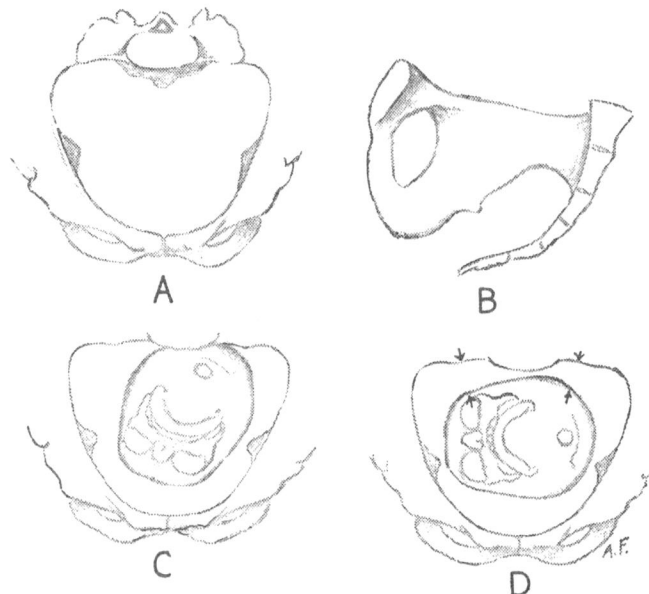

Figure 47.   The mechanism of arrest in the occipitoposterior position
in android types with slight convergence. A, Inlet view to show the shape
of the inlet with slight narrowing of the forepelvis and slight convergence
of the side walls. B, Lateral view. C, Arrest in the occipitoposterior position at midpelvis. The shape of the pelvis aids in causing this position.
D, The flat posterior pelvis prevents rotation of the ovoid head beyond
the transverse position. From this position the delivery is usually terminated by Barton forceps as shown in Fig. 44.

Arrest in the posterior position at midpelvis in anthropoid
forms was treated by several different mechanisms. The most
successful maneuvers followed the principle that in anthropoid
types the head should be brought to lower levels, with its long
axis favoring the long anteroposterior pelvic diameters and
avoiding the narrow transverse diameters of the pelvis.

This principle may be carried out by the pelvic application
of pelvic curved forceps with traction to lower levels followed
by complete anterior rotation on the pelvic floor (Fig. 49). As
a rule, convergence of the side walls is present to hinder an-

terior rotation at the level of arrest. Descent to lower levels in the posterior position as illustrated in Fig. 49 should not be attempted if the sacrum is forward. We found one case in which the forward sacrum was fractured between the third and fourth sacral segments when this mechanism was forcibly employed. In one instance, in an extreme anthropoid pelvis, the child was delivered face to pubis.

Manual rotation to the anterior position at the level of arrest may be employed without difficulty if the pelvis is ample

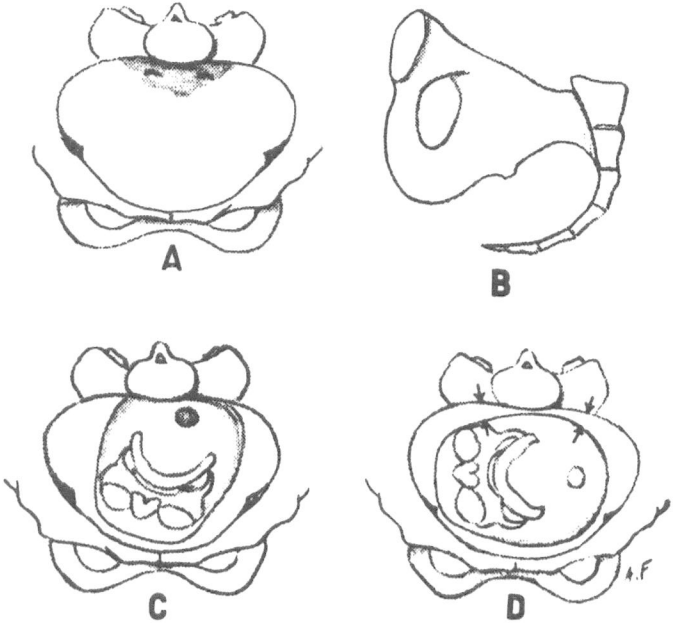

Figure 48. The mechanism of arrest in the occipitoposterior position in flat types with a backward sacrum. A, Inlet view. B, Lateral view to show the backward inclination to the sacrum with increased sacral concavity into which the occiput rotates. C, Arrest in the occipitoposterior position in midpelvis. D, As in the android type, Fig. 47, the posterior pelvis prevents rotation of the ovoid head beyond the transverse position. From this position delivery is usually terminated by the use of Barton forceps as illustrated in Fig. 44.

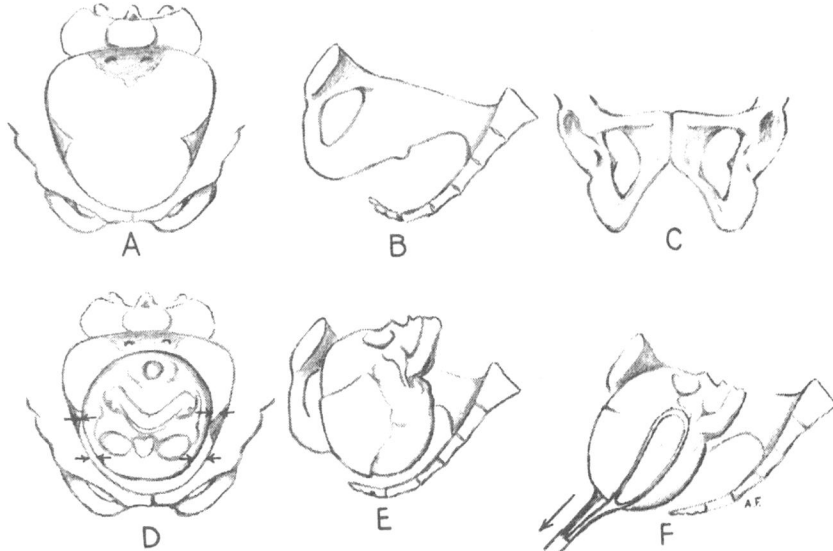

Figure 49. The mechanism for delivery from arrest in the occipito-posterior position to lower levels in the same position. A, Android-anthropoid type of pelvis with a long anteroposterior diameter, prominent ischial spines, and converging side walls. B, Lateral view to show ample posterior pelvic capacity because of an average curvature and inclination to the sacrum. C, Anteroposterior view of the slightly narrowed subpubic arch. D, Arrest in the occipitoposterior position, inlet view. E, Arrest in the occipitoposterior position, lateral view. F, A pelvic application of pelvic curved forceps is made and traction exerted downward and forward. A low complete rotation may be accomplished with caput in sight.

in width at the ischial spines, but is usually more successful if performed at a higher level in the spacious upper pelvis.

The complete rotation of a posterior position by forceps or the "Scanzoni" maneuver is seldom used in midpelvic arrest in the posterior position. When successful, the child is usually small and the head reveals good flexion and molding. This maneuver is rarely successful when there is significant restriction in transverse diameters as occurs in extreme anthropoid types. In fact, it is not mechanically advisable to rotate through a narrower diameter a head which has adjusted itself to a longer diameter. The same objection applied to the use of the transverse mechanisms as described for the android and flat types of pelvis (Figs. 47, 48). In a few instances, the head was rotated to the transverse position in certain anthropoid types and delivered to lower levels in this position before anterior rotation was performed. Apparently the success of the maneuver was due to the ample transverse diameters of the anthropoid-gynecoid or gynecoid-anthropoid types. In cases of extreme anthropoid pelves, however, the child would be subjected to the possibility of serious injury by encouraging descent in the transverse position.

Low Midpelvic Arrest in the Posterior Position

The posterior position is a physiologic position for the anthropoid type of pelvis, as shown by the higher incidence of this type in cases of low and low midpelvic arrest. Android and flat forms are rarely associated with the posterior position at low levels. The investigation revealed another fact which has been clinically substantiated, namely, that manual and instrumental methods of rotation are more successful for posterior positions arrested low in the pelvis than for those at higher levels. From the standpoint of the pelvis alone, this is difficult to explain as the typical anthropoid pelvis with posterior arrest usually shows definite restriction in transverse diameters throughout the mid and lower pelvis. It was pointed out in case of midpelvic arrest that forced rotation in midpelvis through a narrow diameter may be hazardous after the head has become adjusted to the long sagittal diameter of the anthropoid types. The same principle holds for low arrest in the posterior position, but the danger is less here because of good flexion and molding on the part of the head. The significance of the abnormal pelvis in many respects is modified by the degree of flexion and molding of the head.

Complete manual rotation may be successfully carried out if arrest has occurred in the forepelvis with the head bulging the pelvic floor, but this success depends on the presence of at least moderate transverse diameters in the interspinous and intertuberous regions. Complete anterior rotation by forceps or the "Scanzoni" maneuver is also more successful at this low level than at the midpelvis. If resistance to the act of rotation is encountered, forceful efforts should not be employed because transverse diameters may be more restricted than was anticipated. Although the use of pelvic curved forceps applied in the reverse cephalic position is advised by most obstetricians, Kielland forceps have been found most efficient for this maneuver.

If resistance to either manual or instrumental anterior rotation is encountered at this low level, the head may be elevated and the rotation performed at higher levels. One stillbirth occurred because this maneuver was not used until after forceful efforts had been employed at the level of arrest with caput in sight (Fig. 50). The child was seriously injured by repeated attempts at manual and instrumental methods of rotation. The pelvis conformed to an extreme anthropoid-android type with marked restriction in transverse diameters throughout the pelvis. The head was easily rotated after it was elevated to the inlet. From this position it descended to the pelvic floor and was delivered by low forceps. This particular patient has subsequently had a spontaneous delivery of an average sized child, face to pubis.

Face-to-pubis delivery may be encouraged occasionally if the lower sacrum does not obstruct, and is sometimes less hazardous than forceful efforts at rotation. Usually low rotation can be accomplished after the head has been brought slightly downward and forward in the direct posterior position. This may avoid the deep perineal lacerations which frequently attend an instrumental face-to-pubis delivery.

The method used commonly for flat and android forms in midpelvic arrest in the occipitoposterior position (i.e., manual rotation to the transverse with application of forceps, lateral

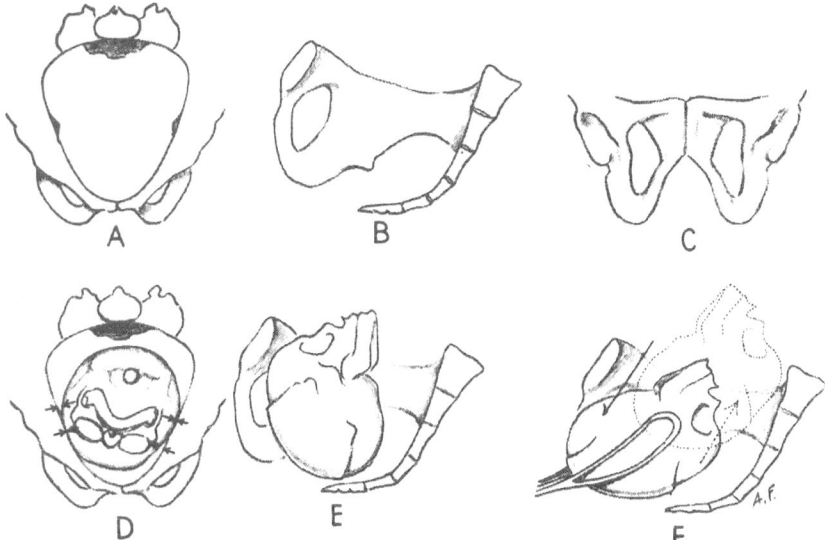

Figure 50. The mechanism of elevation with high manual rotation in extreme anthropoid types. A, Inlet view showing a long anteroposterior diameter with marked transverse narrowing throughout the pelvis. B, Lateral view indicating a slightly forward lower sacrum. C, Anteroposterior view of the narrow subpubic arch. D, Arrest in the occipitoposterior position in the lower forepelvis with caput in sight. Attempts at anterior rotation at the level of arrest were unsuccessful because of the restriction in transverse diameters. These attempts at rotation seriously injured the child, causing a stillbirth. E, Lateral view of arrest in the occipitoposterior position. F, Delivery was finally accomplished easily by elevation of the head toward the inlet followed by manual anterior rotation at this high level. The head rapidly descended to the outlet where low forceps were applied.

flexion, and descent to the pelvic floor with low anterior rotation) was rarely employed at this low level.

Summary of Occipitoposterior Arrest of the Head

Arrest of the head in midpelvis in the occipitoposterior position is most frequently associated with two pelvic types—the ample android type with slight convergence and the flat type with a backward sacrum. These latter two factors (convergence or backward sacrum) create ample anteroposterior space in the midpelvis to allow the occiput to rotate posteriorly. Incomplete flexion and molding of the head favor the maneuver of manual rotation of the head to the transverse position with the application of Barton forceps followed by lateral flexion and descent with low rotation. Arrest in more characteristic anthropoid forms has been successfully treated by utilizing the ample sagittal diameters as is done by the pelvic application of forceps to the occipitoposterior position with descent to a lower level and rotation with caput in sight. A Scanzoni maneuver was rarely used at the level of arrest and was successful only with a small child in an ample anthropoid form.

In the low medium arrest of the head in the occipitoposterior position the number of characteristic anthropoid forms increases. Maximum flexion and molding of the head allowed more success with complete rotation by manual or instrumental methods than occurred with arrest at a higher level.

The methods of treatment for arrest in the posterior position discussed above, and related to the type of pelvis which favors each particular mechanism, may be listed as follows:

1. Manual anterior rotation at level of arrest.
2. Elevation of the head followed by manual anterior rotation (Fig. 50).
3. Delivery to the pelvic floor in the posterior position followed by low complete rotation (Fig. 49).
4. Face-to-pubis delivery.
5. Scanzoni maneuver.
6. Manual rotation to the transverse with descent to pelvic floor followed by low anterior rotation (Figs. 47, 48).
7. Anterior spiral rotation with descent.

TREATMENT OF ARREST IN THE ANTERIOR POSITION

Arrest in the anterior position, as with the posterior position, is associated with two common architectural features, i.e., an ample anteroposterior diameter and converging side walls with a decrease in the interspinous diameter. A cephalic application of forceps is easily made and the degree of traction necessary to effect delivery is, to a certain extent, dependent upon the degree of convergence of the side walls. The widest biparietal diameter of the head descends through the intertuberous diameter in front of the narrowed interspinous diameter.

THE PELVIC OUTLET AS INFLUENCED BY LOWER SACRAL VARIATIONS

Convergence of the side walls and variations in sacral curvature and inclination may effect a change in pelvic shape at and below the level of the ischial spines. The importance of convergence of the side walls has been repeatedly stressed in a discussion of the mechanism of forceps deliveries in the android and anthropoid types.

In the sagittal plane, variations in the curvature and inclination of the sacrum affect the relationship of the lower sacrum and sacrococcygeal platform to the ischial spines and change the shape of the pelvic outlet. The frequency with which the forward sacrum was noted in the low medium and medium forceps groups shows the influence that restriction of posterior outlet space plays in pelvic arrest. An attempt has been made to illustrate the common types of lower sacral variation by the use of suitably chosen case studies.

In Fig. 51, A–C, the lower sacrum curved forward to a considerable degree below the level of the ischial spines. The long posterior sagittal diameter at the level of the spines and the generally large pelvis allowed rapid descent until the head was arrested by the forward sacral tip. The shape of the outlet has been converted into a flat transverse oval which necessitates the delivery of the head to a lower level in the transverse position by forceps as illustrated.

In the example shown in Figure 51, D–F, a somewhat simi-

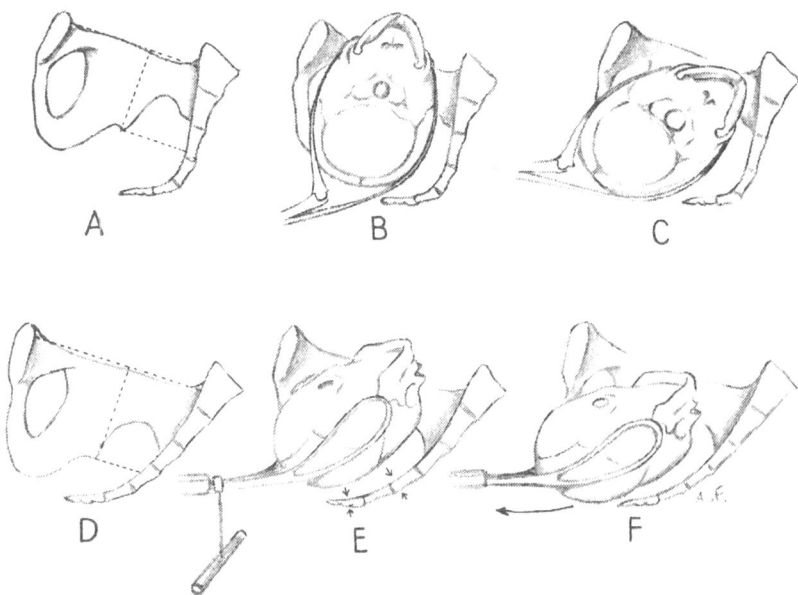

Figure 51. Significance of sacral variations. A, Lateral view of a large anthropoid pelvis with a forward lower sacrum. The posterior sagittal diameter at the level of the spines is long. The sacrococcygeal platform is elevated toward the level of the spines. The sacral tip and coccyx extend forward under the spines, causing a short anteroposterior diameter at the outlet and a flat outlet shape. B, Arrest of the head in the transverse position on the sacrococcygeal platform. The posterior parietal bone is depressed. C, Barton forceps were easily applied. The head was flexed laterally toward the outlet and anterior rotation was accomplished after the biparietal diameter had passed the sacral tip. D, Lateral view of an ample flat type of pelvis with good sacral concavity and forward lower sacral tip. Same pelvis as illustrated in Fig. 17, D. E, Arrest of the large head occurred on the sacrococcygeal platform close to the sacrum. The good sacral concavity allowed descent to this level. F, Barton forceps brought the head close to the pubic rami by lateral flexion. With traction, force was misdirected against the symphysis. Barton forceps were removed and pelvic curved forceps were applied in cephalic application. The head easily descended by downward and forward traction. Anterior rotation occurred after the biparietal diameter of the head had passed the sacral tip.

lar shape existed at the outlet. The pelvis conformed to a large flat type which predisposes to a transverse arrest. The good sacral concavity and ample posterior sagittal diameter at the level of the spines allowed the head to descend to be arrested by the forward sacral tip. It was necessary to deliver the head in the transverse position through the forepelvis until the biparietal diameter had passed the sacral tip before anterior rotation could be obtained. Barton forceps were used to flex laterally the head over the pelvic outlet close to the pubic rami. Barton forceps, however, failed to bring about descent because force, with traction, was misdirected against the pubic rami. After a cephalic application was obtained by pelvic curved forceps, the correct axis of traction was determined, and the head descended in the direction indicated in the diagram (Fig. 51, D–F).

The example shown in Fig. 52, A–C, reveals the significance of increased posterior outlet space caused by a straight sacrum with a slightly backward inclination. The pelvis, an android-flat type, allowed the head to descend in the R.O.T.–R.O.P. position until the posterior aspects of the perineum began to bulge. The shape of the pelvis prevented rotation but the adequate posterior pelvic shape caused by the straight backward sacrum allowed this low descent. The patient was delivered by low forceps. Barton forceps brought about anterior lateral flexion, and anterior rotation was easily accomplished with caput in sight.

The influence of the forward sacral inclination is shown in Fig. 52, D–F. The head was arrested in the direct anteroposterior position on the pelvic floor. Attempts at delivery with pelvic curved forceps failed when traction was exerted downward and backward. Force was misdirected against the forward sacrum. As soon as an attempt was made to extend the head, descent and an easy delivery occurred.

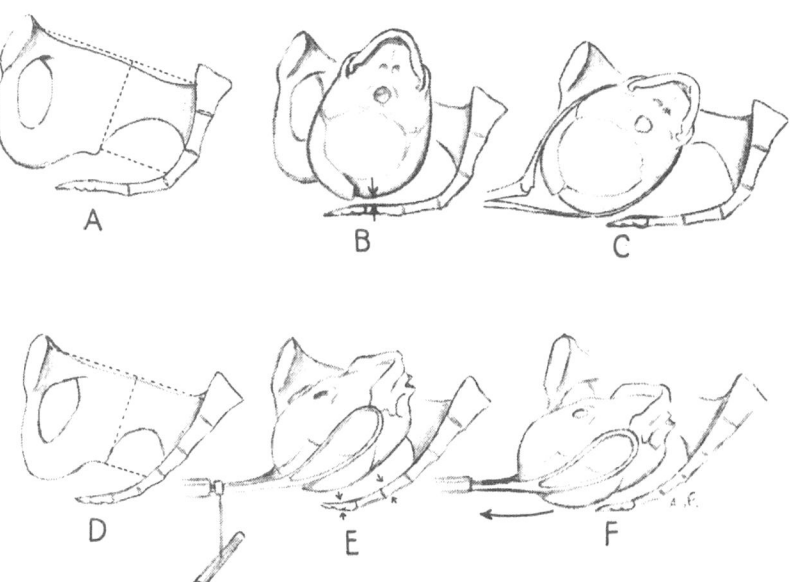

Figure 52. Significance of sacral variations. A, Lateral view of a flat android type of pelvis. The sacrum is straight with a slight backward inclination. The long posterior sagittal diameter at the level of the spines and the straight sacrum presented no obstruction to the descent of the head. Arrest occurred on the pelvic floor in the O.P.–O.T. position because the shape of the pelvis prevented anterior rotation. (Same pelvis as illustrated in Fig. 17, B.) B, Lateral view of arrest with Barton forceps applied. C, Lateral flexion with forceps removed the influence of the posterior pelvis and allowed anterior rotation. D, Lateral view of the ample anthropoid type with a forward inclination to the sacrum. (Same pelvis as illustrated in Fig. 17, C.) E, Arrest occurred just above the pelvic floor in the oblique anterior position because of the forward sacrum. Haig Ferguson forceps were applied. A downward and backward traction caused no advance of the head because traction force was misdirected against the lower sacrum. F, Elevation of the handles of the forceps caused slight extension of the head and with a downward and forward axis of traction descent occurred easily.

Section V

Recognition of Disproportion

DISPROPORTION between the fetus and the amount of space available in the bony pelvis varies considerably in degree. In the great majority of patients nature has provided a comfortable margin for the fetus, so that large women will often bear normally large children easily, while small women bear normally small children just as easily. In certain cases, however, the fetus is too large for the pelvis regardless of the type of the pelvis. In other cases the shape of the pelvis is such that the space available for the child is reduced to a serious degree even though the various cardinal diameters may be of normal size.

Disproportion has long been considered in two categories: absolute and relative. The criteria for these categories have varied with time. Playfair,[14] in 1865, discussing indications for cesarean section, describes absolute disproportion as existing when the pelvis is so small as to prevent delivery of the child through it even by destructive operations. Later, absolute disproportion was held to exist when the child could not be born *alive* through the pelvis. At present, there are many who consider that absolute disproportion exists when the child cannot be delivered *safely* through the pelvis. Relative disproportion, on the other hand, has long been held to exist when there was enough room for the child to be delivered through the pelvis by some obstetric maneuver, although the natural forces were

95

not sufficient to produce delivery. To this has been added the consideration that it must not only be possible to deliver the child, but the procedure must be safe for the child.

It becomes imperative, then, to recognize the presence of disproportion. This is a continuing process during the course of the pregnancy, and consists of the following steps:

1. Clinical examination of the pelvis, with classification of the shape, estimation of the size, and a tentative prognosis.

2. Observation late in pregnancy for size of child and expected engagement near term.

3. Reexamination clinically at the onset of labor.

4. Trial of labor.

5. Estimation of disproportion by x-ray pelvimetry.

Step 1. In early pregnancy it is seldom possible to forecast the possibility of disproportion with great accuracy. Disproportion is a problem compounded of pelvis, child, and labor; and it is only when the pelvis is very small, or greatly deformed, that a confident prediction of serious disproportion can be made. In this regard it is noteworthy that there have been 3 patients at the Sloane Hospital for Women with a true conjugate at the inlet of 8 cm who have been delivered easily from below, and at term, of normal, albeit small, children. At the other extreme is a patient with a true conjugate of 13 cm who required cesarean section after a hard trial of labor, the baby being extremely large. The chief value of the early clinical examination is thus to alert the physician to the statistical probability of trouble in that particular patient. It is unusual indeed to encounter difficulty with the gynecoid pelvis, unless the child is very large. The flat pelvis is relatively rare, but it too produces difficulty only when the true conjugate is markedly shortened. The anthropoid pelvis, on the other hand, will be associated with a difficult labor in about 20 per cent of cases, the usual difficulty being a persistent posterior position. The android pelvis, worst of all, is associated with difficulty in some 40 per cent of cases, with serious disproportion at the inlet or the mid-pelvis being not uncommon. When the pelvis is anything other than gynecoid, it would be of advantage to obtain an expert opinion and, perhaps, x-rays before labor has begun.

Step 2. As the end of pregnancy approaches the size of the child can be estimated, not too accurately it must be admitted, but well enough to decide whether a small, average or large child is present. Two weeks before term, in the usual primigravida, the head should engage. A pelvic or rectal examination done at this time should reveal the tip of the head at the level of the ischial spines, and should produce a definite impression of the relative size of head and pelvis.

Step 3. Complete examination of the patient early in labor should include abdominal and rectal examinations. If the head is not definitely engaged, a pelvic examination with full sterile technic will allow a final clinical estimate of the relation of the size and position of the child to the size and shape of the pelvis. Unless the head is engaged, and unless the impression of ample space is gained, x-ray examination of the patient should be carried out.

Step 4. A trial of labor may be decided upon with or without x-ray examination, and is certainly indicated in the great majority of patients. Elective cesarean section should be performed for disproportion only in those cases where an accurate technic of pelvimetry has revealed a dangerously high degree of disproportion. The trial of labor, carried out with careful attention to mother and child, can be stopped when it is clear that no further progress is being made, and cesarean section can be carried out with no greater risk than that of elective cesarean section. It is often gratifying to observe an apparently high degree of disproportion, as measured clinically, overcome easily and safely by good labor. On the other hand, it is unwise to persist in the trial of labor where severe disproportion is clearly shown to exist by x-ray. For this reason, all patients undergoing trial of labor should have x-ray pelvimetry, and the films should be studied by the physician performing the delivery in every case.

X-RAY PELVIMETRY

X-ray pelvimetry should be performed only in those cases in which clinical evidence of disproportion exists. The incidence will vary from one location to another, depending upon population types, but even in teaching institutions it should probably not exceed 10 per cent.

The time at which the films are obtained is of some importance. The purpose of the films is to determine the relationship of the bony parts at the time of delivery, and the problem ought, therefore, to be studied as close to the time of delivery as possible. This means that most films should be taken after the onset of labor. When films are taken before labor there are several disadvantages. First of all, the dates may be wrong, and a long time may elapse before labor occurs. It will then become necessary to take at least one more film to remeasure the size of the head. Second, the position of the head is often unfavorable before the onset of labor. Various attitudes are seen, many of which make measurement of the head questionable, so that a repeat film will be necessary subsequently. The only cases in which x-ray pelvimetry should be performed before the onset of labor are those in which the likelihood of elective cesarean section seems very large.

Technical Considerations

There is required a technic of x-ray pelvimetry which will do two things. First, it must allow accurate measurement of all of the diameters desired. Second, it must show the true shape of the pelvis, particularly the inlet, so that the effect of shape upon the diameters can be determined. There are at least twenty-three technics which allow a reasonably accurate measure of the various diameters. The accuracy should be plus or minus 2 mm. Many technics, however, although simple and accurate as far as measurement of the diameters is concerned, do not show the true shape of the inlet. It is therefore necessary to become more elaborate, and to use a method which shows the true shape of the inlet, either a positioning method or a stereoscopic method.

X-ray pelvimetry has been carried out at the Sloane Hospital for more than 40 years during which time over 16,000 cases have been studied. The stereoscopic method of Caldwell and Moloy, the Ball method, the Colcher–Sussman method, and various modifications of these have been used and on the basis of this experience it is possible to state that there is no one single best technique. Study of films taken using these methods led to the demonstration by Caldwell and Moloy that the shape of the pelvis is an important factor in determining its capacity. In 1938 Moloy proposed that the capacity of the inlet might be measured by fitting a circle into the inlet as it was viewed in the stereoscope or on a flat film. A method for estimating disproportion based on this concept was subsequently described.[18]

The desirable technic of x-ray pelvimetry, then, will be one of several which will allow measurement of diameters and which will also allow a circle to be fitted to the inlet. Pelvic capacity can then be measured. The size of the fetal head can next be measured. Clinical estimation of the size of the fetus is notoriously misleading. It has been shown that while there is a general correlation between the size of the baby's head and the weight of the baby, the extremes of variation may be very large[19, 20, 21] (Fig. 53). In the group of babies with a biparietal diameter of 9.5 to 9.9 cm, the smallest child weighed 1,900 grams and the largest weighed 5,000 grams. It becomes important to measure the size of the head. This can be done quite readily and with considerable accuracy in vertex presentations, although the breech presentation presents very real difficulties. The head may be measured in the precision stereoscope with a consistent accuracy of plus or minus 2 mm. However, the head can also be measured in the standing lateral film. The accuracy of examination in this film was pointed out by Rohan Williams,[22] who, in a study of babies delivered by elective cesarean section, determined that the

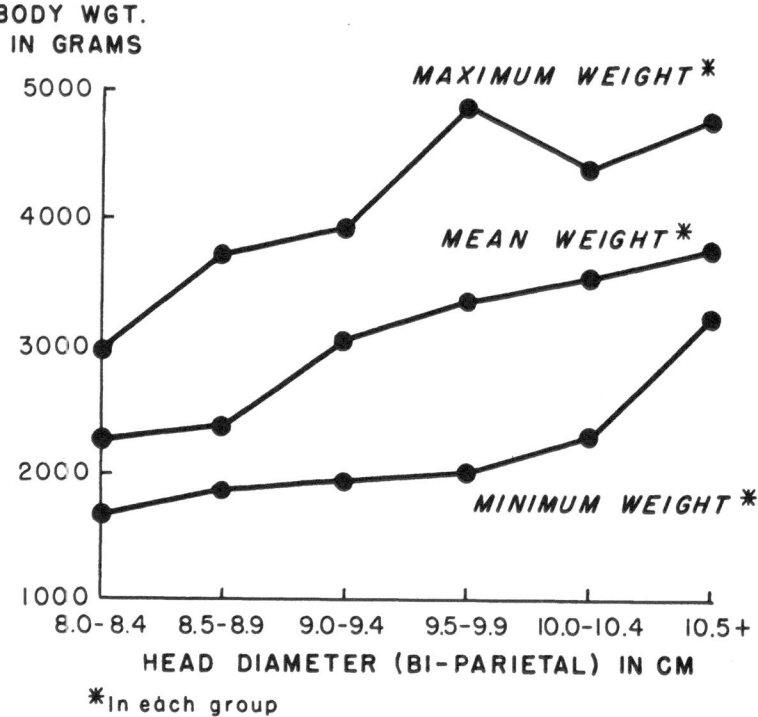

Figure 53. Relation between head size and body weight in the newborn.

error in measurement of the head (except in those rare in-stances when the head was seen in a grossly distorted view) was the same as for the measurements of the pelvic diameters. Thus, in any simple technic which allows measurement of the pelvic diameters in the lateral view the head may also be meas-ured. The size of the head may then be correlated with the size of the pelvic diameters and with the amount of space available as determined by the use of a circular form.

Details of Technic

Standard x-ray equipment with a tube-film distance of 40 inches and a Potter-Bucky diaphragm with a 16:1 grid is used for the standing anteroposterior and lateral films. This apparatus may also be used for stereoscopic films if precision stereoscopy by the Caldwell-Moloy method is not to be performed. If the Caldwell-Moloy method is used, it is necessary to use a tube-film distance of 25 inches and an 8:1 grid.

An anteroposterior film in the upright position is taken. A lateral film with the patient standing is next taken, the patient turning 90 degrees to her right from the position in which the anteroposterior film was taken. A metal ruler is placed between the buttocks for the lateral view.[23]

The patient is then placed supine on the table, and a pair of stereoscopic views are taken, with a tube shift of 2½ inches, the target being centered at the level of the anterior superior iliac spines. When precision stereoscopy is to be carried out, the technic described by Moloy[15] is used.

When simple stereoscopy is desired, the cassette markers and the triangular markers are omitted, and any convenient tube-film distance is used. A triangular sponge rubber pad about 5 inches high is placed under the lumbosacral area. This causes the pelvis to flex backward into such a position that the inlet is parallel, or nearly parallel to the films. These films can then be viewed stereoscopically (although no measurements can be made in the stereoscope) or they can be viewed as flat films if desired.

A remark about stereoscopy is necessary at this point. It is important to view stereoscopic films in such a way that the distance from the eye to the film is the same as the distance from the target of the x-ray tube to the film at the time the films were taken. If different distances are used, a "stereoscopic" image can always be obtained, but this image will be distorted. The observer will not be aware of this distortion, for the image seems to be a good one. It was the accidental discovery of this fact which led to the development of the "precision stereoscope" with its close attention to detail. When precision stereoscopy is used, it is necessary to have the eye-film distance exactly the same as the tube-film distance, and the special markers used in the Caldwell-Moloy technic make this possible. But when ordinary stereoscopy is to be carried out it is necessary to have the eye-film distance within 3 cm of the tube-film distance, otherwise the image of the pelvis will be distorted and misleading.

Method of Reading Films

The anteroposterior and lateral films are examined in the standard viewing box. The stereoscopic films are examined in the stereoscope, or, when it is seen that the inlet is parallel to the film, one of the stereoscopic films can be examined as a flat film in the standard viewing box. The data are gathered according to a prepared work sheet (Table 4). The films are

TABLE 4.   FORM FOR REPORTING PELVIMETRY FILMS

The senior house officer is responsible for this.
The following scheme should be used:
  1. Give patient's name and x-ray number.
  2. "X-ray pelvimetry reveals a . . . . pelvis with the
     following measurements:
        AP of inlet . . . . cm
        Widest transverse of inlet . . . . cm
        Circle of inlet . . . . cm
        Interspinous diameter . . . . cm
     The diameter of the fetal head is . . . . cm
     The side walls are (straight, convergent, divergent).
     The sacrum is (straight, curved) and has a (forward, average, backward)
        inclination.
     The distance from the tip of the sacrum to the coronal plane through the
        spines is . . . . cm
     The subpubic arch is (wide, average, narrow)
     The fetus presents by the (vertex, breech, etc.) in the . . . .
        position, with the leading part at . . . . station.
     The difference at the inlet is . . . . cm
     The difference at the spines is . . . . cm
     This represents (no, borderline, absolute) disproportion.
                        Report by Dr. . . . .
     This scheme may be varied as necessary, but the *pelvic type* and the *measurements* should always be given.

---

first examined generally, all of the bony structures seen being checked for congenital or other anomalies, and for symmetry. The obstetrical presentation and position are noted. The type of the pelvis is determined according to the Caldwell-Moloy classification.

Measurements are made as follows:

1. In the standing lateral film (Fig. 54):

    A. The anteroposterior diameter of the inlet is found by following the somewhat boat-shaped shadows produced by the flare of the ilia at the pelvic brim, and a line (A–A) is drawn at the level of the inlet from the posterior aspect of the symphyis to the anterior aspect of the sacrum. The promontory of the sacrum is seldom in the obstetrical inlet. The curve of the posterior part of the inlet generally sweeps into the first or second sacral vertebra. Anteriorly, the superior surface of the body of the pubis rises somewhat above the general

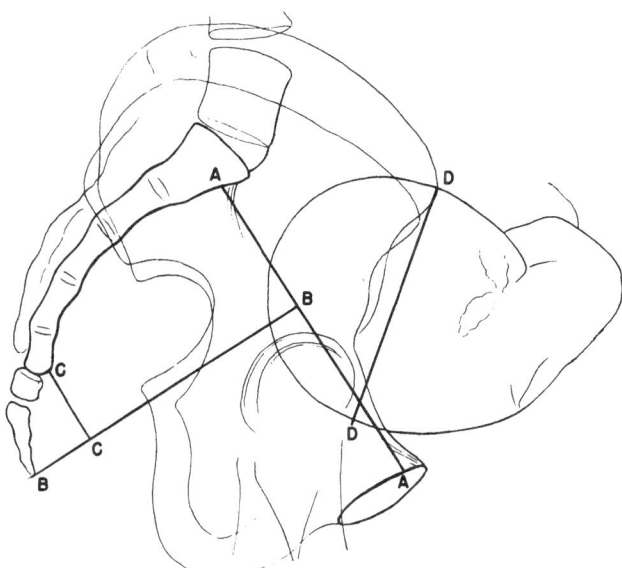

Figure 54. Method of measuring the standing lateral film.

level of the inlet proper, so that the anterior edge of
the true inlet lies about 1 cm below the top of the
symphysis.

B. The positions of the spines are marked, and a point
   midway between the spines is taken. A line (B–B) is
   then dropped through this point perpendicular to the
   line of the inlet, and extending caudad beyond the tip
   of the sacrum. This line represents the coronal plane
   through the spines. The intersection of this line and
   the line of the inlet (A–A) locates the position of the
   widest transverse diameter of the inlet.

C. A line (C–C) is then drawn from the tip of the sacrum, parallel to the line of the inlet, and intersecting
   the coronal plane through the spines.

D. The fetal head is next examined (in vertex presentations) and a line (D–D) is drawn in the plane of the
   suboccipitobregmatic and biparietal diameters. In 20
   per cent of cases one or the other of these diameters
   will be clearly seen, the fetal head being found in the
   direct occipitoanterior, occipitoposterior, or occipito-
   transverse position. In 80 per cent of cases the head
   will be rotated to some extent away from these direct
   positions. In the great majority of cases, this rotation
   will be a simple one around the long axis of the head.
   In this event, the plane of the biparietal and suboccipitobregmatic diameters is readily recognized and
   measurement of the diameter as seen on the film is carried out. When the measurement of this diameter is
   compared with the actual value of the biparietal diameter it is found that the measured diameter is either
   equal to the biparietal or larger by not more than 3
   mm. Occasionally the head is rotated in a more complex manner. In this event, it is not possible to identify
   the plane of the biparietal diameter, for the complex
   rotation brings an oblique frontoccipital diameter into
   profile. When this type of shadow is seen, measure-

ment should not be carried out. Fortunately, this type of rotation is very rare when films are taken after the onset of labor.

The length of the anteroposterior diameter (A–A) and of the diameter of the fetal skull (D–D) are measured with a ruler. These measurements are then corrected by using the buttocks marker, which is marked in centimeters. Since these diameters are in the same plane as the marker, the distortion will be equal, and a simple count of centimeters will give the true diameter.

The length of the line C–C is measured directly on the film, and no correction is made. This distance is generally small, and variations of the amount introduced by correction are not clinically significant.

It should be noted that the position of the patient must be close to a pure lateral if measurements are to be made. With the tube centered at the left greater trochanter, a "perfect" lateral will result when the sacrosciatic notches are superimposed. If the peaks of these notches are more than 1 cm apart the readings may be questioned, and if they are more than 2 cm apart measurements should not be made.

2. The standing anteroposterior view (Fig. 55):
    E. The widest transverse diameter of the inlet is drawn by inspection, E–E. The actual length of this diameter is then calculated according to the method described by Ball. This diameter lies at the point of intersection of the plane of the inlet and the coronal plane through the spines. This point is seen on the lateral film (intersection of A and B). The distance from this point to the outer margin of the sacral shadow is measured, along a line parallel to the posterior edge of the film. The outer margin of the sacrum represents the anterior face of the cassette holder, and the film is actually 4 cm. beyond this face. The distance from the point of

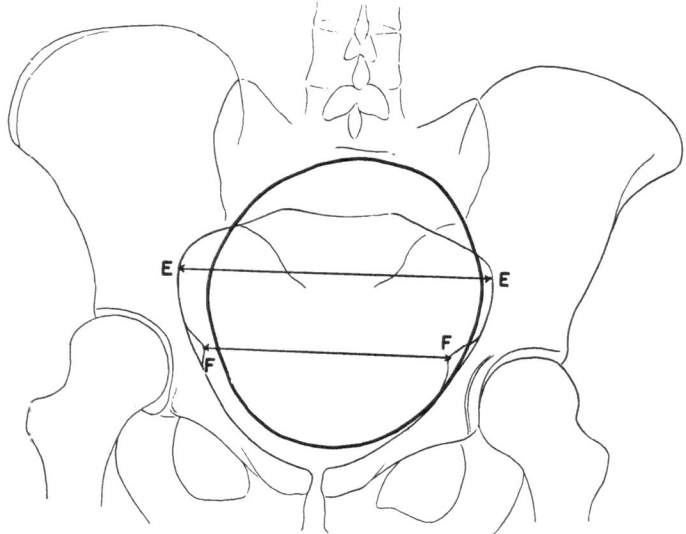

Figure 55.   Method of measuring the standing anteroposterior film.

intersection of lines A and B to the outer margin of
the sacrum, plus 4 cm, represents the distance from
the widest transverse diameter of the inlet to the film.
Since the tube-film distance is already known, it is possible to set up an equation by which the true value of
the diameter can be determined.*

F. The interspinous diameter, F–F, is then measured. The
true value of this diameter is calculated by the same
method described for the widest transverse diameter
of the inlet, with the point between the spines on the

---

* There are two aids to this calculation, the nomogram described by
Ball,[16] and the special slide rule devised by Schwarz.[24] In addition, the
use of a 40 inch tube film distance makes this very easy. This distance is
100 cm, nearly enough, so that the object-film distance at once allows
a percentage to be established. Thus, if the distance from the widest
transverse diameter to the outer shadow of the sacrum is 13 cm, and
the depth of the film holder is 4 cm, the "object-film" distance will be
17 cm. The ratio of the true diameter to measured diameter according
to the rule of similar triangles will then be 100 − 17/100, or 83/100, or
83 per cent.

lateral film used as the position of the interspinous diameter.

3. The stereoscopic films:

When the precision stereoscope is available, the antero-posterior diameter of the inlet, the widest transverse diameter of the inlet, the interspinous diameter, the circle of the inlet, and the diameter of the fetal head can all be determined by the method described by Moloy and Steer.[4]

When the precision technic is not available, the stereoscopic films must be taken with the inlet parallel to the film, or a flat film should be taken with the inlet parallel to the film. The purpose of the stereoscopic or of this special flat film is to determine the influence of the shape of the pelvis upon the space available to the head. The simplest and most effective method of doing this is to place a circular disk (cut out of cardboard) in the inlet. This is

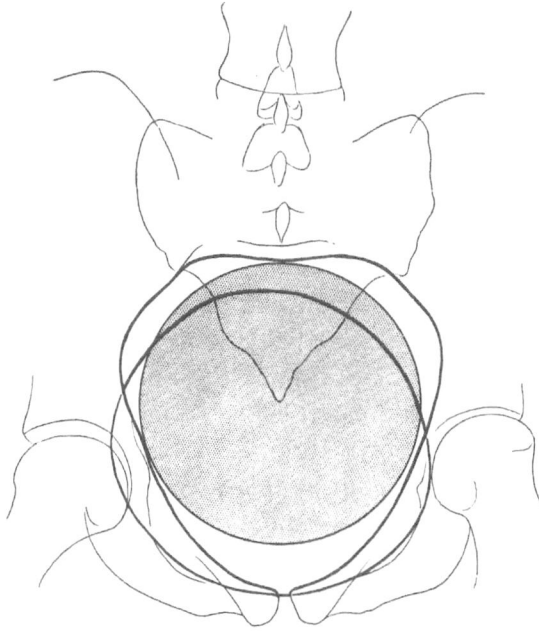

Figure 56. Method of placing a circle in the pelvic inlet.

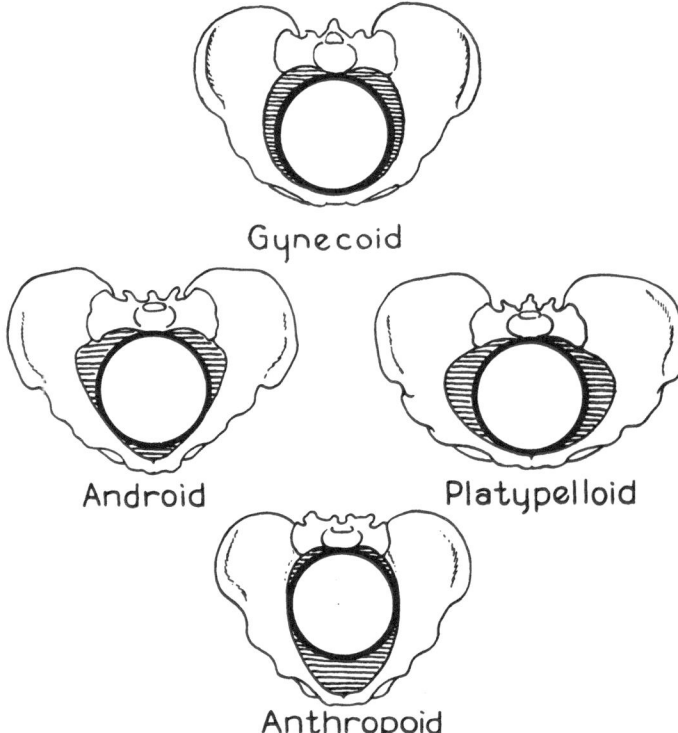

Gynecoid

Android   Platypelloid

Anthropoid

Figure 57.   Diagrams to show how a circle fits each of the four pure
types at the inlet.

done with great ease in a properly taken flat film, and the
effect of shape is readily apparent (see Figs. 56 & 57).
The actual size of this circle is equal to the anteroposterior
diameter in gynecoid and flat pelves, but is smaller than
this diameter in android and anthropoid pelves. When a
circle is found which just fits the inlet, its true diameter
can be readily calculated. The true anteroposterior diameter is already known from the lateral view. A ratio can
then be set up as follows: measured AP diameter on "flat"
film/true AP diameter = measured diameter of circle/true
diameter of circle.

It is obvious that other technics may be used to determine the true diameters listed above, but it is most im-

portant that the diameter of a circle which fits the inlet always be determined.

Estimation of Disproportion

The possibility of disproportion is then estimated. The diameter of the head is subtracted from the diameter of the circle which fits the inlet. The numerical difference between these two diameters is called the "difference at the inlet," and this is the index of disproportion at this level.

The diameter of the head is next subtracted from the interspinous diameter. This number is the "difference at the spines." This produces an index of disproportion at the interspinous diameter, but this must be considered in relation to the amount of space before and behind the interspinous diameter. It is not possible to fit a circle into the plane of the spines. Two other factors are therefore considered here: the degree of forwardness of the sacrum* (line C–C in the lateral film), and the width of the subpubic arch.† A special film of the arch may be taken if desired, but the clinical description is adequate.

* The forwardness of the sacrum: The measurement described above (line C–C) is the result of a number of attempts to measure the anteroposterior diameter at the level of the spines. The anterior rim of the plane through the spines extends out into space under the subpubic arch, the distance being a function of the arch. Measurements of the anteroposterior diameter from the sacrum to the arch have been made. Measurements from various points on the sacrum to the inferior aspect of the symphysis, and to the anterior end of the anteroposterior diameter of the inlet, have been made. These have been correlated with the outcome of labor by themselves. They have been related to the size of the head in various ways, and these results have been correlated with the outcome of labor. None of these correlations have worked out as well as the simple one of measuring the distance from the tip of the sacrum to the coronal plane through the spines.

† The subpubic arch: Measurement of the bituberous diameter, of the angle of the arch, of the depth of the arch (from the inferior aspect of the symphysis to the bituberous diameter) and of various combinations of these have been made. These have been correlated with the outcome of labor. The "measurement" which gives the best correlation is the simple description of the arch as "narrow" or "not narrow," and this description works as effectively when made by clinical examination as when made by x-ray.

INTERPRETATION OF X-RAY FINDINGS

Long experience, and careful correlation of the outcome of labor in various types of cases, has demonstrated that a strictly accurate prognosis can never be given in the individual case from the x-rays alone, except in those extremely rare instances of gross pelvic distortion. When very high degrees of disproportion are present, some patients will still be delivered from below, because of great molding and powerful labor. When no disproportion is present some patients will still require operative delivery because of faulty position or attitude, or because of poor labor. X-ray examination provides a statistical statement of the probability of serious arrest in the individual case, and this can then be used as one factor in determining the best method of delivery. When one speaks of "accuracy" of x-ray prognosis, it is important to define the type of prognosis. If a "yes or no" prognosis is desired, x-rays are of no value. But if an accurate statistical prognosis is desired, the described method of x-ray study will provide it. The soundness of the figures stating the "probability of serious arrest" was tested by making this study in 3 steps. The first 350 cases were totaled, then another 300, and finally the remaining 986. The percentages in each subgroup agreed within 0.5 per cent, so that the figures for the entire group represent consistent findings.

CORRELATION OF X-RAY PROGNOSIS WITH OUTCOME OF LABOR

In order to determine how accurately the outcome of labor may be forecast by means of x-ray pelvimetry, it is necessary to study only the cases in which an adequate trial of labor has been given. This excludes cases of elective cesarean section, and cesarean section performed with insufficient labor. It excludes cases of cesarean section or of forceps delivery performed because of uterine inertia, fetal distress, or other complications. The study group therefore includes all cases of spontaneous delivery, all of "elective" forceps, all of indicated forceps, and all cesarean sections performed after an adequate trial of labor.

Ideally, a trial of labor consists of full dilation of the cervix for 2 hours, with ruptured membranes and with good contractions. Practically, many patients do not reach this point, and therefore a trial of labor is defined as labor which finally results in cessation of progress as measured by the dilation of the cervix and descent of the head. There will be some difference of opinion as to the adequacy of a trial of labor under these conditions, but in each case those responsible for the clinical management of the patient were satisfied that an adequate trial had been given. Where there was any doubt, the case was not used.

DISPROPORTION AT THE INLET

The degree of disproportion at the inlet is expressed as the difference between the diameter of the circle which fits the inlet and the diameter of the fetal head. This difference is correlated with the outcome of labor according to the following groups: 1.0 cm or less, 1.1 cm to 1.4 cm, 1.5 cm to 1.7 cm, and 1.8 cm or greater. The results of this correlation are shown in Table 5.

TABLE 5.   RELATION BETWEEN THE "DIFFERENCE AT THE INLET" AND THE OUTCOME OF LABOR

| | Difference at Inlet | | | | | | | |
| | 1.0 cm or Less | | 1.1 cm to 1.4 cm | | 1.5 cm to 1.7 cm | | 1.8 cm or More | | |
Type of Delivery	No.	%	No.	%	No.	%	No.	%	Total
Spontaneous	15	11	39	28	72	38	422	39	548
Low forceps	12	8	32	23	64	34	627	55	735
Midforceps	7	5	8	6	28	15	48	4	91
Cesarean section	107	76	62	43	25	13	18	2	212
Total	141		141		189		1,115		1,586

It is apparent that some patients (24 per cent) will be delivered from below even in the group with the highest degree of disproportion (difference 1.0 cm or less). Such a high degree of disproportion can be overcome only by extreme degrees of molding, and this may be dangerous to the fetus. In 34 cases of delivery from below, 8 babies were lost because of laceration of the tentorium, a perinatal mortality of 24 per cent. In 107 deliveries by cesarean section, 2 babies were lost. One of these had had a trial at forceps, and died of a lacerated tentorium; and one died apparently of shock though no laceration of the tentorium was found.

It is also apparent that some patients will require cesarean section even when there is no disproportion at the inlet (difference 1.8 cm or greater), because of disproportion below the inlet.

When the difference at the inlet was greater than 1.0 cm there was no perinatal mortality due to the trial of labor, as long as no attempt at forceps delivery was made.

It is possible therefore to state the likelihood of delivery from below with any given degree of disproportion at the inlet, but it is not possible to state the prognosis absolutely in any individual case.

DISPROPORTION AT THE MIDPELVIS

The three indices of disproportion in the midpelvis are considered separately and together. The criterion for disproportion in this group is arrest in the midpelvis sufficient to warrant midforceps delivery or cesarean section. In recent years, cesarean section has been used more freely with midpelvic arrest, not because delivery from below is impossible but because the risk to the child is greater with a difficult forceps delivery than with cesarean section. The method of delivery will necessarily vary from one case to another and under varying circumstances, but the important feature is that the head became arrested in the midpelvis.

TABLE 6. RELATION BETWEEN THE "DIFFERENCE AT THE SPINES" AND THE OUTCOME OF LABOR

	Difference at Spines						
	<0 cm		0-1.0 cm		>1 cm		
Type of Delivery	No.	%	No.	%	No.	%	Total
Spontaneous	27	29	170	27	351	41	548
Low forceps	21	22	275	43	439	51	735
Midforceps	9	10	57	9	25	3	91
Cesarean section	37	39	134	21	41	5	212
Total	94		636		856		1,586

The Difference at the Spines

The difference between the interspinous diameter and the biparietal diameter of the fetus is correlated with the outcome of labor as shown in Table 6. Since arrest in the midpelvis is treated by midforceps and by cesarean section, it is useful to compare the probability of these two types of delivery with that of spontaneous and low forceps delivery. When this is done, the "probability of serious arrest" is obtained. The table shows that the "probability of serious arrest" is 49 per cent when the difference at the spines is less than 0; 30 per cent when the difference is 0 to 1.0 cm; and 8 per cent when the difference exceeds 1.0 cm.

It is significant that the probability of arrest is only 49 per cent even when the biparietal diameter is larger than the interspinous. This is so because of variations in the amount of space present in front of and behind the interspinous diameter itself.

The Distance From the Coronal Plane Through the Spines to the Tip of the Sacrum (CP → S)

This measurement (C–C in Fig. 1) is correlated with the outcome of labor in Table 7. When the incidence of mid-

Table 7.   Relation Between the Distance From the
Coronal Plane Through the Spines to the Tip of
the Sacrum (CP→S) and the Outcome of Labor

	CP → S						
	<3.0 cm		*3.0-4.5 cm*		*>4.5 cm*		
Type of Delivery	*No.*	*%*	*No.*	*%*	*No.*	*%*	*Total*
Spontaneous	52	24	217	31	279	41	548
Low forceps	86	40	315	45	334	49	735
Midforceps	35	17	45	7	11	2	91
Cesarean section	40	19	116	17	56	8	212
Total	213		693		680		1,586

forceps is added to that of cesarean section, the "probability of serious arrest" is seen to vary with CP → S as follows: CP → S less than 3.0 cm, probability of serious arrest 36 per cent; CP → S 3.0 to 4.5 cm, probability of serious arrest 24 per cent; CP → S greater than 4.5 cm, probability of serious arrest 10 per cent. This measurement, it must be noted, is considered as an independent one, without reference to the size of the head or the remainder of the pelvis. In arriving at the complete prognosis, these other factors must be considered also, as is shown below.

The Subpubic Arch

The size of the subpubic arch is correlated with the outcome of labor in Table 8. The probability of serious arrest is seen to vary as follows: subpubic arch narrow, probability of serious arrest 46 per cent; subpubic arch average, probability of serious arrest 13 per cent; subpubic arch wide, probability of serious arrest 17 per cent. This measurement, like the preceding one, is also considered independently here, but in making the final prognosis all of the other features of the pelvis must be considered.

TABLE 8. RELATION BETWEEN THE SIZE OF THE SUBPUBIC ARCH
AND THE OUTCOME OF LABOR

	Subpubic Arch						
	Narrow		Average		Wide		
Type of Delivery	No.	%	No.	%	No.	%	Total
Spontaneous	43	15	411	39	94	38	548
Low forceps	116	39	506	48	113	45	735
Midforceps	28	10	47	5	16	7	91
Cesarean section	103	36	84	8	25	10	212
Total	290		1,048		248		1,586

The Midpelvis as a Whole

In the preceding sections, it has been demonstrated that the probability of serious arrest is greatest when: (1) the difference at the spines is less than 0 cm (probability 49 per cent), (2) the distance from the coronal plane through the spines to the tip of the sacrum is less than 3.0 cm. (probability 36 per cent), and (3) the subpubic arch is narrow (probability 46 per cent). A combination of all 3 of these factors represents the most severe degree of disproportion to be found in the midpelvis. This combination was found in 29 cases. Of these, none were delivered spontaneously; 10 required low forceps, 9 midforceps, and 10 cesarean section. The probability of serious arrest is therefore 65 per cent. However, there were 3 fetal deaths due to birth trauma in this group, 2 with low forceps and 1 with midforceps. The risk to the fetus in delivery from below with this type of disproportion is 3 in 19, or 16 per cent. These infants died of laceration of the tentorium. Descent of the head in this type of case occurs only when there is considerable molding, and the addition of a small amount of force will add enough molding to cause the tentorium to be torn.

MISCELLANEOUS TYPES OF DISPROPORTION

1. *Inlet Disproportion Alone.* There was disproportion at the inlet alone, without any evidence of disproportion in the lower pelvis, in 45 cases. The outcome of labor in these cases is shown in Table 9. The probability of serious arrest was 40 per cent.

TABLE 9.   OUTCOME OF LABOR WITH DISPROPORTION PRESENT
ONLY AT THE INLET

Type of Delivery	Difference at Inlet			
	1.0 cm or less	1.1 cm to 1.4 cm	1.5 cm to 1.7 cm	Total
Spontaneous	3	7	3	13
Low forceps	1	5	8	14
Midforceps	1	5	6	12
Cesarean section	4	2	0	6
Total	9	19	17	45

2. *Difference at the Spines 1 cm or Less.* With no other evidence of disproportion, this occurred in 26 cases, in 9 of which delivery was spontaneous, 10 by low forceps, and 7 by midforceps. There were no cesarean sections. The probability of serious arrest was 27 per cent.

3. *Inlet Disproportion, and a Difference at the Spines of 1 cm or Less.* These were present in 58 cases, in 18 of which delivery was spontaneous, 15 by low forceps, 5 by midforceps, and 20 by cesarean section. The probability of serious arrest was 43 per cent.

4. *Difference at the Spines of 1 cm or Less and CP → S 3.0 cm or Less.* This occurred in 19 cases, 3 with spontaneous delivery, 9 by low forceps, 6 by midforceps, and one by cesarean section. The probability of serious arrest was 37 per cent.

5. *Inlet Disproportion, Difference at the Spines of 1.0 cm or Less, and CP → S 3.0 cm or Less.* These were present in

19 cases, 4 with spontaneous delivery, 4 by low forceps, 2 by midforceps, and 9 by cesarean section. The probability of serious arrest was 58 per cent.

6. *Difference at the Spines of 1.0 cm or Less, and Subpubic Arch Narrow.* These were present in 17 cases, 3 with spontaneous delivery, 10 by low forceps, 3 by midforceps, and one by cesarean section. The probability of serious arrest was 24 per cent.

7. *Difference at the Spines of 1 cm or Less, Arch Narrow, and Inlet Disproportion.* These were present in 20 cases, 4 with spontaneous delivery, 3 by low forceps, one by midforceps, and 12 by cesarean section. The probability of serious arrest was 65 per cent.

8. *Outlet Disproportion.* The pelvic outlet is formed by the ischial tuberosities and the tip of the sacrum. The tuberosities are never involved in bony arrest, because the head comes into contact with the descending rami of the pubes before it reaches the tuberosities in the cases in which the arch is narrowed. The tip of the sacrum can cause arrest in certain instances. Usually the forward tip of the sacrum is a part of generalized pelvic narrowing, so that the arrest is also caused in part by the spines and the descending rami of the pubes. There are cases, however, in which the entire pelvis is adequate except for a forward sacral tip, the head being held against the inferior aspect of the symphysis by the tip of the sacrum. These cases are rare, there being 8 in this series of 1,586. Delivery occurred spontaneously in one of these, by low forceps in 5, and by midforceps in 2. There were no cesarean sections.

9. *The Narrow Subpubic Arch.* All of the features of the pelvis which can cause disproportion can be found occurring alone, except for the narrow subpubic arch. The arch is the easiest part of the pelvis to examine clinically, and it is highly significant that if the arch is found to be narrow there will always be additional features contributing to disproportion.

BREECH PRESENTATION

The estimation of disproportion in a breech presentation is difficult because of two factors. First, it is possible to measure the head accurately in only 9 out of 10 cases, and it is possible to discover which measurement was in error only *after* delivery has occurred. This is so because the unengaged and unfixed head is able to move between films (or during them) and it does move in certain cases. Second, the estimation of degrees of disproportion in a vertex presentation is based upon large numbers of cases in which delivery was carried out from below in the presence of various degrees of disproportion, and such data do not exist for breech presentations. Cesarean section has long been used in these cases, and although from time to time very difficult cases have been delivered from below the numbers of these are too small to be statistically valuable.

For these reasons, a study of breech delivery was undertaken by Todd and Steer using the criterion of *safe* delivery, that is, the fetus alive and uninjured, as indicating *no* disproportion. The pelvis was then measured as though for a vertex delivery, and the shape was described. It was found that if the AP diameter of the inlet is 11 cm or greater, *and* the widest transverse diameter of the inlet is 12 cm or greater, *and* there is no restriction in any of the characteristics of the pelvis, "safe" delivery will occur. It should be noted that this refers to the adequacy of the pelvis in relation to the size of the baby only, and does not pertain to the other hazards of breech delivery such as extended arms, prolapsed cord, and so on. It was obvious in the cases studied that management of these complications was easier and more effective when the pelvis was adequate. In this study, it was also found that steady progress in cervical dilation and descent of the presenting part was associated with safe delivery. It is a sign of "fetopelvic" disproportion when arrest of labor takes place in the presence of an "adequate" bony pelvis. Stimulation of labor with oxytocics, or attemps at manual procedures to assist delivery from below under these circumstances is dangerous. It may be noted that in this series a cesarean section rate of 30 per cent with breech presentations was justified.

It should be noted that the x-ray films provide additional information of value in cases of breech presentation. The type of breech (frank, footling, etc.), the degree of flexion or extension of the vertebral column, the position of the arms, and particularly the degree of extension of the head may influence the labor and delivery, and may dictate cesarean section in certain cases when the pelvis is found to be "adequate."

VALUE OF THE X-RAY DATA

The value of such prognostic data is to allow a consideration of the entire case with a clear idea of what type of delivery will probably be necessary. These data will allow a recommendation of elective cesarean section only in one group—the group in which the difference at the inlet is 1.0 cm or less. Even this recommendation is not based on the impossibility of delivery from below with this degree of disproportion, for 24 per cent of these patients will be delivered from below. It is based upon two facts: (1) that 76 per cent will require cesarean section, and (2) that the perinatal mortality in this group is 23 per cent when delivery does occur from below. Thus the x-ray findings even in this degree of disproportion are closely related to the clinical features of the case.

Since this is the only group of cases in which the x-ray finding is of paramount importance, all other cases should be given a trial of labor. The method of conducting this trial of labor will vary with the statistical prognosis as given by x-ray examination. A very long trial of labor will obviously not be carried out in the face of a high degree of disproportion. On the other hand, demonstration of the absence of disproportion will allow a long trial of labor and, if necessary, the use of drugs to stimulate the labor. Forceps delivery, when progress has stopped, can be carried out with a detailed description of the disproportion available, and cesarean section can be used instead of forceps when the degree of disproportion is demonstrated to be great.

The technic of x-ray pelvimetry is thus shown by this study to be an important aid in the management of labor, but, except for one very small group of cases, it is not the prime factor upon which the decision as to type of delivery should be made.

References

1. Derry, D. E.: On the sexual and racial characteristics of the human ilium. J. Anat. & Physiol., 58:71, 1923.
2. Turner, W.: The index of the pelvic brim as a basis of classification. J. Anat. & Physiol., 20:125, 1885–86.
3. Thoms, H.: Newer aspects of pelvimetry. Am. J. Surg., 35:372–378, 1937.
4. Smith, G. E., and Jones, F. Wood: The Archaeological Survey of Nubia. Report for 1907–08, Vol. 2, p. 1910.
5. Caldwell, W. E., and Moloy, H. C.: Anatomical variations in the female pelvis and their effect in labor with a suggested classification. Am. J. Obst. & Gynec., 26:479, 1933.
6. Caldwell, W. E., Moloy, H. C., and D'Esopo, D. Anthony: Further studies on the pelvic architecture. Am. J. Obst. & Gynec., 28:482–497, 1934.
7. Caldwell, W. E., Moloy, H. C., and D'Esopo, D. Anthony: The more recent conceptions of the pelvic architecture. Am. J. Obst. & Gynec., 40:558–565, 1940.
8. Schuman, W. A.: A new measurement (clinical) for estimating the depth of the true pelvis. Am. J. Obst. & Gynec., 28:497–500, 1934.
9. Denman, Thomas: An Introduction to the Practice of Midwifery. New York, G. & C. & H. Carvill, 1829.
10. Holland, E. A.: Report on Public Health. Great Britain Ministry of Health, 1922, No. 7.
11. Moloy, H. C.: Studies on head molding during labor. Am. J. Obst. & Gynec., 44:762–782, 1942.
12. Fabre and Trillat: Contributions a l'étude du détroit superieur dans le bassin normal par la radiographie métrique. Bull. Soc. d'obst. et de gynec. de Par., 2:707–714, 1913.
13. Thoms, H.: The type of pelvis intimately associated with occipito-posterior position. Surg., Gynec. & Obst., 56:97–100, 1933.

14. Playfair, W. S.: A Handbook of Obstetric Operations. H. Renshaw, London, 1865.
15. Moloy, H. C.: A new method of roentgen pelvimetry; preliminary report. Am. J. Roentgenol. *30*:111–114, 1933.
16. Ball, R. P., and Marchbanks, S. S.: Roentgen pelvimetry and fetal cephalometry: new technic; preliminary report. Radiology, *24:* 77–84, 1935.
17. Colcher, A. E., and Sussman, W.: Practical technique for roentgen pelvimetry with new positioning. Am. J. Roentgenol. *51:*207–214, 1944.
18. Moloy, H. C., and Steer, C. M.: New method of quantitative estimation of cephalopelvic disproportion. Am. J. Obst. & Gynec., *60:* 1135–1146, 1950.
19. Ince, J. G. H.: On value of cephalometry in estimation of foetal weight. J. Obst. & Gynaec. Brit. Emp., *46:*1003–1010, 1939.
20. Donaldson, S. W., and Cheney, W. D.: Prenatal estimation of birth weight by pelvicephalometry. Radiology, *50:*666–672, 1948.
21. Kosar, W. P., and Steer, C. M.: Relation of body weight to biparietal diameter in newborn. Am. J. Obst. & Gynec., *71:*1232–1235, 1956.
22. Williams, E. R.: Radiologic diagnosis of disproportion. Brit. J. Radiol., *16:*173–181, 1943.
23. Weitzner, S. F.: Simple roentgenographic method for accurately determining true conjugate diameter of pelvis. Am. J. Obst. & Gynec., *30:*126–128, 1935.
24. Schwartz, G. S.: Simplified method of correcting roentgenographic measurements of maternal pelvis and fetal skull. Am. J. Roentgenol., *71:*115–120, 1954.

Index